Local, Regional, and Free Flaps for Head and Neck Reconstruction

Rod Rezaee • Akina Tamaki
Editors

Local, Regional, and Free Flaps for Head and Neck Reconstruction

Basics and Foundations

Springer

Editors
Rod Rezaee, MD
Ear, Nose and Throat Institute
University Hospitals Cleveland
Medical Center
Cleveland, OH, USA

Case Western Reserve University School
of Medicine
Cleveland, OH, USA

Akina Tamaki, MD
Ear, Nose and Throat Institute
University Hospitals Cleveland
Medical Center
Cleveland, OH, USA

Case Western Reserve University School
of Medicine
Cleveland, OH, USA

Department of Otolaryngology- Head
and Neck Surgery
Lewis Katz School of Medicine at
Temple University
Philadelphia, PA, USA

ISBN 978-3-032-03210-2 ISBN 978-3-032-03211-9 (eBook)
https://doi.org/10.1007/978-3-032-03211-9

This Springer imprint is published by the registered company Springer Nature Switzerland AG
The registered company address is: Gewerbestrasse 11, 6330 Cham, Switzerland

To:

My late father M. Hassan Rezaee, MD, without whose unwavering confidence in me, encouragement, motivation, and tireless work ethic, I would not have been given the opportunity to write this text. He modeled dedication to his patients, friends, and family, a model that has served me well to emulate. Thank you, Dad.
A successful career in Head and Neck Surgery and Microvascular reconstruction involves the support of many individuals. I am fortunate to have had many who devoted time, energy, knowledge, humor, advice, and guidance along the way. I view it as each holding a piece of the puzzle. Without that piece, the picture would not be complete.

I thank:

My mentors who provided the inspiration to pursue this path.
My colleagues, fellows, residents, and students who challenge me to bring my best daily.
My nursing and staff partners who provide the necessary team care before, during, and after surgery, without whom successful outcomes in microvascular surgery are not possible.
My patients and their families, for having faith in me and giving me the privilege of caring for them.
My family, mom, and sisters who give me love, joy, and an ear to listen.
My sons, Grayson and Benjamin, who give me perspective, purpose, and wonder each day.
My wife, Sara, whose love and support have been present since this journey began and would not have been possible or complete without her.

Rod Rezaee, MD

To:

My parents, Keiichi and Masako, who have supported me in all my goals and throughout all my endeavors.
My sister, Fumi, whom I admire so much and to whom I owe much of my success.
My husband, Berje, for his love and help in making our partnership greater than the sum of its parts.
I dedicate this book to our daughter, Rika, who has brought indescribable joy to my life.

Akina Tamaki, MD

Preface

Head and Neck Reconstruction is an endeavor that demands labor, emotion, and time. The field has evolved immensely in the more than 30 years since my medical education and training began. The complexity of the problems patients, and therefore we as their surgeons, face has increased dramatically, mandating we evolve as a discipline together to meet these ever-changing demands. New types and increased complexity of grafts have been developed and refined, skill and outcomes have improved, and teams have formed around patients, pushing surgical and reconstructive boundaries forward over those three decades. While technically demanding and often intense procedures, the reward comes in the form of sharing the outcomes with our patients, the optimal and suboptimal, enjoying the former with them, and learning from the latter to improve for the next time.

The goal of this book is not to provide an exhaustive text of Head and Neck Reconstruction, but rather a concise, yet complete, collection of the myriad of local, regional, and microvascular free flaps available to the reconstructive surgeon, be they a student, resident, fellow, or attending in the fields of Otolaryngology-Head and Neck, Plastic, or Oral Maxillofacial Surgery. The authors have been selected for their expertise, and we thank them for their time and effort to provide clear descriptions of the procedures to include relevant anatomy, pearls, pitfalls, and surgical steps. The text is not meant to replace mastering surgical anatomy, which serves as the foundation of a successful surgery and outcome. Please use it as a study guide, a review, a reliable and insightful reference, and use it to expand options available to you as you face defects brought on by cancer ablation, trauma, or congenital anomalies.

The field of Head and Neck Reconstruction is one of the greatest disciplines available to pursue and one that offers an incredible opportunity to improve the quality of life for patients. With continued thought, study, and collaboration, the field will continue to evolve over time, resulting in new flap designs, improved surgical techniques and patient outcomes, and, most importantly, renewed and improved hope for the patients under our care. Thank you for your time and interest.

Cleveland, OH, USA | Rod Rezaee, MD

Contents

Part I

Local and Regional Flaps

1 Cervicofacial Flap

Humzah Quereshy and Nithin S. Peddireddy

History

- Introduced in the literature by Esser in 1918 [1] as a cheek rotational flap; its current modern iteration using both advancement and rotation modifications was introduced by Juri and Juri in 1979 [2].

Indications and Benefits

- Reconstruction of soft tissue defects of the cheek, brow, temple, ear, and orbit.
- Can be used primarily for closure of defects or in combination with other rotational or microvascular free tissue flaps.
- Shorter operative time with reduced anesthetic and surgical resource needs when used primarily.
- No additional donor site wound, second team, or microvascular instrument needs.

H. Quereshy
Ear, Nose and Throat Institute, University Hospitals Cleveland Medical Center, Cleveland, OH, USA

Case Western Reserve University School of Medicine, Cleveland, OH, USA

N. S. Peddireddy (✉)
Department of Otolaryngology- Head and Neck Surgery, Karmanos Cancer Center, Detroit, MI, USA
e-mail: peddireddyni@karmanos.org

Anatomy

- The cervicofacial flap incorporates portions of both the cheek and the neck.
- Neck layers include the skin, subcutaneous tissue, and platysma.
- Cheek layers include the skin, subcutaneous tissue, and superficial musculoaponeurotic system (SMAS).
- The facial nerve is deep to the SMAS and platysma. It is crucial to know the layer to protect the nerve during harvest.
- Vascular supply is based on random arterial and venous supply via the subdermal plexus [3].
  - Arterial supply includes tributaries/perforators from the facial, submental, superficial temporal (via orbito-zygomatic branch), transverse cervical, preauricular, and superior thyroid arteries.
  - Venous supply is irregular and drains into both anterior and external jugular veins.

Preoperative Care

- Perform a comprehensive head and neck exam. Focus on evaluation for prior scars, trauma, and skin laxity.
- Obtain comprehensive surgical and medical history, including history of radiation.
- Counsel patient on the anticipated defect in the context of facial subunits and the potential

R. Rezaee, A. Tamaki (eds.), *Local, Regional, and Free Flaps for Head and Neck Reconstruction*,
https://doi.org/10.1007/978-3-032-03211-9_1

for secondary distortion that may result once the flap is inset (i.e., the eye and the risk of ectropion).
- Discuss smoking preoperatively and counsel tobacco cessation perioperatively. Active smokers have a higher risk of complications including flap failure [4].

Special Instruments and Positioning

- Consider facial nerve monitoring or clinical monitoring of the nerve.
- Can be performed under local anesthesia.
- Ensure a wide surgical prep to incorporate pectoral, deltoid, as well as the posterior neck depending on anticipated defect size and location.

Modifications

- Incorporation of deltopectoral tissue.
- Can be elevated in a subplatysmal/sub-SMAS vs subcutaneous plane. This enables bulkier myocutaneous flaps with vascular supply from branches of the facial artery [5].
- Can be used for cutaneous coverage in combination with rotational myogenous flaps such as pectoralis/temporal/trapezius flaps or with microvascular free tissue transfers when external resurfacing is needed and to optimize color/tissue match and aesthetic outcome.
- Tissue expanders can also be considered to allow for larger skin defects to be amenable for repair with a cervicofacial flap [6].

Pitfalls and Complications

- Risk of distal tip necrosis and wound dehiscence due to random blood supply of tissue in the distal aspect of the flap.
- Risk of facial nerve injury. This is often transient, and initial management should be conservative.
- Ectropion can result if flap extends superiorly near the orbit causing inferior traction or scarring.

Postoperative Care

- Can consider head and neck flexion to reduce tension on the flap.
- Placement of postoperative drain in inferior neck to reduce hematoma risk. Remove after 2–5 days based on output.
- Standard incisional care with topical ointments until wound is healed.
- If the incision extends close to the eye, would recommend local eye care. This includes ophthalmic ointments or consideration of tarsorrhaphy in select cases. Additional support sutures of the flap and soft tissue resuspension to minimize downward pull can be considered.

Tissue type: *Fasciocutaneous, myocutaneous*
Artery: *Subdermal plexus*
Vein: *Subdermal plexus, contributions from the anterior and external jugular vein*
Nerve: *None*
Flap reach: *Can reach superiorly to the supraorbital margin, laterally to the postauricular area, and medially to the midline*
Flap size: *Variable depending on skin laxity and locations chosen to recruit skin*

Operative Procedure

1. Design incision in a relaxed skin tension line posterior from the defect for an anterior-based flap or inferior for a posterior-based flap. If necessary, can remove skin around the defect to allow for more cosmetic closure. In addition, wide undermining around the defect can be of benefit for closure and to minimize size of defect to repair (Fig. 1.1) [8–11].

   * Pay special attention to critical structures such as the eye or nose to prevent ectropion or nasal obstruction and distortion.
2. If no medical contraindication, widely inject dose appropriate local anesthetic with vaso-

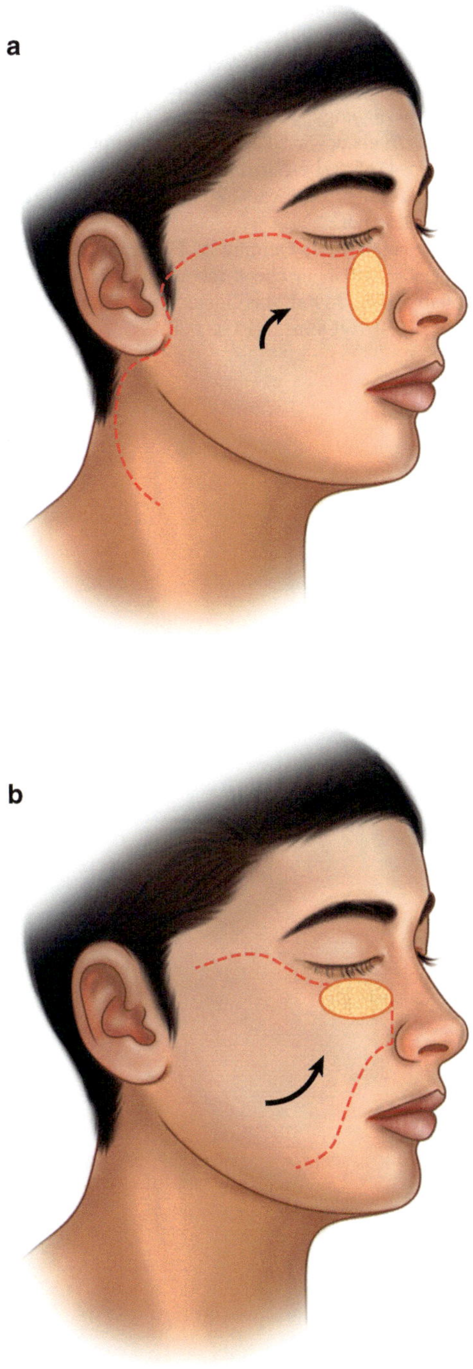

Fig. 1.1 (**a**) Anteriorly-based cervicofacial flap—anteromedial rotation for a medial defect with a longer vertical dimension; (**b**) posteriorly-based cervicofacial flap—posterosuperior rotation for superior defect with a longer horizontal dimension

constrictor (1% lidocaine with 1:100,000 epinephrine) in the face and neck.

3. Incise through skin and subcutaneous tissue in the face or neck.

   * Can consider a subplatysmal/sub-SMAS elevation.

4. Flap is elevated from distal to proximally. During this elevation, the flap is frequently evaluated and brought toward the defect to determine the size of flap needed and to identify areas of tethering where further flap elevation or release is necessary.
5. Once there is adequate tissue to cover the defect, attention is turned to the standing cone deformities that are created surrounding the defect. If possible, it is ideal to camouflage this in a relaxed skin tension line. Care must be taken to not narrow the base of the flap when addressing standing tissue cones with Burrow's triangle tissue excision.
6. Meticulous hemostasis is then achieved, and suction drains are placed.
7. A layered closure of the neck and face is performed.

   * If necessary, one can place tacking sutures to the periosteum of the orbit to minimize the risk of ectropion and to aid with soft tissue support especially in larger flaps.

Disclosure Statement No conflicts of interest to disclose.

References

1. Esser J. Rotation der Wange. Leipzig: Vogel; 1918.
2. Juri J, Juri C. Advancement and rotation of a large cervicofacial flap for cheek repairs. Plast Reconstr Surg. 1979;5:692–6.
3. Freeland AP, Rogers JH. The vascular supply of the cervical skin with reference to incision planning. Laryngoscope. 1975;85:714–25.
4. Kinsella JB, Rassekh CH, Hokanson JA, Wassmuth ZD, Calhoun KH. Smoking increases facial skin flap complications. Ann Otol Rhinol

Laryngol. 1999;108(2):139–42. https://doi.org/10.1177/000348949910800206.
5. Tan ST, MacKinnon CA. Deep plane cervicofacial flap: a useful and versatile technique in head and neck surgery. Head Neck. 2006;28:46–55.
6. Ashab Yamin MR, Mozafari N, Mozafari M, Razi Z. Reconstructive surgery of extensive face and neck burn scars using tissue expanders. World J Plast Surg. 2015;4(1):40–9.
7. Rhodes R, Moreau A, Romano E, Cannon T. The cervicofacial flap. Oper Tech Otolaryngol. 2019;30:145–50. https://doi.org/10.1016/j.otot.2019.04.010.
8. Kaplan I, Goldwyn RM. The versatility of the laterally based cervicofacial flap for cheek repairs. Plast Reconstr Surg. 1978;61:390–3.
9. Stark RB, Kaplan JM. Rotation flaps, neck to cheek. Plast Reconstr Surg. 1972;50:230–3.
10. Manana W, Fagan J. Cervicofacial flaps in head and neck reconstruction. Open Access Atlas of Otolaryngology, Head & Neck Operative Surgery. https://vula.uct.ac.za/access/content/group/ba5fb1bd-be95-48e5-81be-586fbaeba29d/Cervicofacial%20flaps%20for%20head%20and%20neck%20reconstruction.pdf
11. Al Shetawi AH, Quimby A, Fernandes R. The cervicofacial flap in cheek reconstruction: a guide for flap design. J Oral Maxillofac Surg. 2017; https://doi.org/10.1016/j.joms.2017.08.006.

Deltopectoral Flap

2

Nilam D. Patel and Theodoros N. Teknos

History

- First reported in the literature by Aymard in 1917 for nasal reconstruction and again by Joseph in the 1930s [1, 2].
- Popularized further by Bakamjian [3] in 1965 for pharyngoesophageal defects and was widely utilized until the introduction of musculocutaneous flaps.

Indications and Benefits

- Reconstruction of cutaneous cervical and soft tissue defects including coverage of exposed great vessels and reconstruction of hypopharyngeal or laryngopharyngeal defects.
- Thin and pliable flap with excellent color match to cervicofacial skin.
- Versatility in skin paddle design and size with multiple reliable perforators.
- Minimal donor site morbidity.
- Donor site is outside of typical field of head and neck radiation.
- Can be used in conjunction with a second flap to achieve reconstructive goals.

N. D. Patel · T. N. Teknos (✉)
Ear Nose and Throat Institute, University Hospitals Cleveland Medical Center, Cleveland, OH, USA

Case Western Reserve University School of Medicine, Cleveland, OH, USA
e-mail: theodoros.teknos@UHhospitals.org

Anatomy

- Arterial supply to the upper chest wall is derived from the internal mammary artery (IMA), also referred to as the internal thoracic artery (Fig. 2.1).
- The IMA originates from the first division of the subclavian artery near its origin.
  - IMA runs posteroinferiorly 1 cm lateral to the sternal border bilaterally and gives off 5–6 fasciocutaneous perforators that exit through the intercostal spaces [4].
  - Perforators course laterally and superficially to the fascia overlying the pectoralis major and deltoid muscles.
  - Perforating vessels supply the pectoralis major muscle, soft tissue, and skin medial to the deltopectoral groove.
  - The second and third intercostal perforators are the most robust and, therefore, must be incorporated [4].
  - The diameter of the IMA near its origin is approximately 3 mm and narrows to 1.5 mm at its distal aspect [5].
  - Perforators on average are 0.7 mm in diameter but can vary from 0.5 to 1.2 mm [6].
- Lateral to the deltopectoral groove, arterial supply to the skin overlying the deltoid is randomly based with perfusion dependent on the subdermal plexus from musculocutaneous

R. Rezaee, A. Tamaki (eds.), *Local, Regional, and Free Flaps for Head and Neck Reconstruction*,
https://doi.org/10.1007/978-3-032-03211-9_2

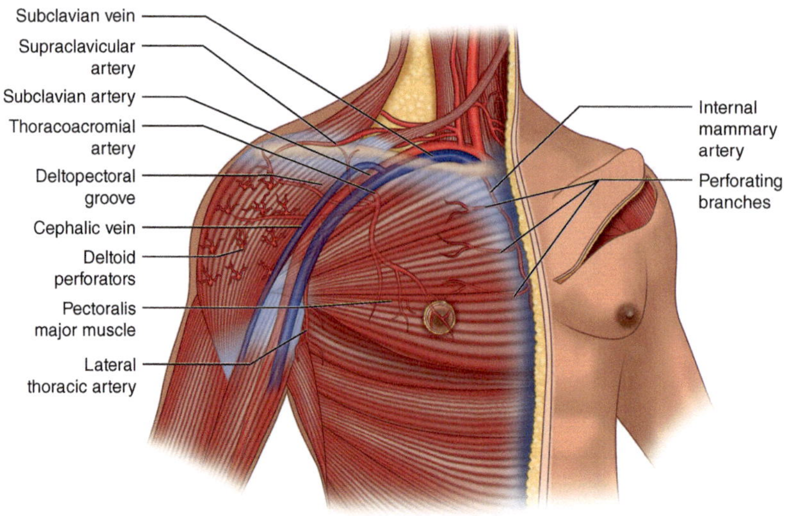

Fig. 2.1 Illustration representing the arterial architecture of the deltopectoral regional flap. The internal mammary artery (IMA) is shown as the first branch off the proximal subclavian artery with IMA perforators extending laterally. Distal to the deltopectoral groove, the random pattern of blood supply via subdermal plexus is shown. A raised left deltopectoral flap is illustrated centered over the IMA perforators

arteries from the underlying deltoid muscle. There are also contributions from the cutaneous branches of the thoracoacromial artery.
  - Transition from the medial axial flap to the lateral randomly based cutaneous flap is marked by the deltopectoral groove, which houses the cephalic vein [7].
  - Medially based flaps are preferred for improved viability and reliability.
- Venous drainage is dependent on the venae comitantes (can be single or double) and the internal mammary vein [5].
- Deltopectoral skin paddle can incorporate tissue spanning between the sternoclavicular joint medially to the deltopectoral groove laterally.
- Cutaneous innervation of the deltopectoral region is via the supraclavicular nerves of C3, C4, and anterolateral intercostal nerves of T2, T3, T4. The anterior chest wall is supplied by anterior branches of intercostal nerves traveling in the intercostal spaces [5].

Preoperative Care

- Assess for history or scars from prior chest wall surgery (e.g., mastectomy) or cardiac surgery that may have harvested the IMA as a bypass vessel.
- Left chest wall utilization may be suboptimal in patients with cardiac disease or those with preexisting cardiac device implants.

Special Instruments and Positioning

- Prepare potential skin graft harvest site as donor site necessitates.

Modifications

- Can be completed as a single-stage or a two-stage reconstruction.
  - The deltopectoral island flap can be harvested by raising subdermal flaps, de-

epithelializing portions of the flap, and tunneling the flap under a bridge of native tissue. This allows for use in single-staged reconstruction.

Can be further modified to be a fascial island flap by de-epithelializing all skin and utilizing the flap for soft tissue reconstruction only.

- Without modifying as an island flap, reconstruction often requires a second-stage for take down of the pedicle and return to donor site.

- A delay procedure is utilized to achieve increased length of the skin paddle by improving survivability of the randomly perfused skin overlying the deltoid.
  - The delayed flap approach is rooted in the angiosome concept. Elevating and severing the musculocutaneous branches overlying the deltoid, while preserving the medial axial arterial pedicle, allows the distal flap to form new blood supply in a more favorable pressure gradient and survive the stress of relocation [6, 7].
  - May be considered when time is available such as elective reconstructions or for post-traumatic defects [8].
  - Can be done with local anesthetic in a clinic setting.
- Internal mammary artery perforator (IMAP) flap.
  - Entails identifying a robust second or third perforator and designing a flap with an associated skin paddle parallel to the intercostal space/perforator.
    - The perforator should be identified superiorly and dissected along its course, the flap is raised in the subfascial plane, islanded, divided laterally, and rotated to cover the defect allowing for primary closure of the harvest site [9].
    - Good for small to medium sized defects of the lower neck/peristomal region and has the benefit of increased arc of rotation.

Pitfalls and Complications

- Poor cosmesis, especially if a skin graft is required.
- Distal flap necrosis is most significant complication seen in up to 17–26% of cases [6, 10].
  - Use of the deltopectoral flap for laryngopharyngeal/hypopharyngeal defects has declined due to the higher risk of distal tip necrosis and ensuing complications.
- Effects of gravity and difficulty in restricting patient neck movement increases risk of distal wound separation.

Postoperative Care

- Apply a bolster or wound vacuum on the split thickness skin graft on the lateral shoulder.
- Physical therapy to the operative shoulder will need to be minimized in the acute postoperative period until skin graft take is confirmed.
- Avoid neck ties and other pressure inducing devices overlying the flap.

Tissue type: *Fasciocutaneous*

Artery: *Perforators originating from internal mammary artery*

Vein: *Venae comitantes from internal mammary vein*

Nerve: *Supraclavicular nerves of C3, C4, and anterolateral intercostal nerves of T2, T3, T4*

Flap reach: *Can reach as far as the preauricular skin or intraorally*

Flap size: *Maximal size varies based on body habitus; however, flaps 20 cm in length × 10 cm in width are reliable. Length can be extended by 6–8 cm with the delay procedure to incorporate the deltoid skin*

Operative Procedure

1. Design the medially based skin flap centered over the second or third intercostal spaces at the sternal border. The base should include at least three to four intercostal spaces to increase the number of perforators. Utilize a

Doppler to identify precise location of perforators during flap design.

* Borders of the skin flap:
  - Superiorly: infraclavicular line.
  - Inferiorly: level of the fifth rib (~10 cm below superior border). An easy way to approximate this is to measure two finger breadths above the male nipple [7].
  - Medially: first four intercostal spaces 2 cm lateral to the sternal border.
  - Laterally: mid-deltoid if planning a delayed procedure, the deltopectoral groove if no delayed procedure is planned.

* Wider flap will limit arc of rotation.

* Plan incision superior in those that may need a pectoralis major myocutaneous flap in the event salvage reconstructive options are needed.

2. Flap is elevated lateral to medial in the subfascial plane. Incise laterally from the skin down to the pectoralis fascia and carefully cut the fascia to expose the underlying muscle. Continue flap elevation medially from the deltoid including the fascia overlying the deltoid and pectoralis muscle. The muscle fibers should be exposed during harvest. Cease elevation at least 2 cm lateral to the sternal border to avoid injury to the main IMA perforators (Fig. 2.1).

   * The lateral perforators from the thoracoacromial artery are sacrificed as they travel through the deltoid and pectoralis major muscles laterally near the deltopectoral groove.

   * IMA perforators emerge 1 cm laterally from the sternal border in the intercostal spaces [7].

   * If performing a delay procedure, cease elevation at the deltopectoral groove and lay the elevated tissue back into place and tack down with sutures. Return in 2–5 weeks, complete elevation as described above.

3. Rotate the elevated skin paddle to cover the defect. Ensure there is no tension or excessive rotation compressing perforators or venous outflow.

   * To improve reach and decrease tension, the flap may be partially de-epithelialized and tunneled under the intervening native skin or, alternatively, that native skin may be sacrificed.

4. The donor site will require closure via split thickness skin graft to cover the lateral shoulder. Apply a compressive bolster or wound vacuum.

   * If planning two-staged reconstruction with the intention of pedicle division in 2–5 weeks, the proximal tissue can ultimately be returned to its native site. The split thickness skin graft will temporarily maintain healthy tissue at the donor site until the pedicle is divided.

Island Flap

1. Design a laterally based skin paddle to maximize reach with the planned pivot location approximately 4 cm from the sternum [11]. Utilize a Doppler to identify the supplying perforators and design the skin paddle centered on this.

   * The skin paddle can be designed lateral to the deltopectoral groove if needed; however, this needs to be done in a delayed fashion. For the delay, incise the lateral aspect of planned skin paddle 270° and elevate the planned skin paddle in a subfascial plane. Tack back down with sutures for a period of 2–5 weeks [12].

   * This can be done locally in clinic to avoid general anesthesia.

2. Incise skin over the midpoint of the pedicle from the planned skin paddle to sternal border. De-epithelialize the skin from the subcutaneous tissue superiorly and inferiorly in a subdermal plane.
3. Elevate the pedicle from the chest wall in a lateral to medial fashion in a subfascial plane and include the skin island. Again, cease elevation 2 cm lateral to the sternal border. Once free, tunnel the flap subcutaneously over the clavicle to reach the defect.
4. The donor site can be closed primarily.

   * De-epithelialized skin can be used to graft the exposed muscle if primary closure is not feasible. Saving this skin can save the patient or reduce the size of a second donor site.

Disclosure Statement No conflicts of interest to disclose.

References

1. Aymard J. Nasal reconstruction. Lancet. 1917;2:888–91.
2. J. J. Nasenplastik und sonstige Gesichtsplastik nebst einem Anhang iiber Mammaplastik und einige weitere Operationen aus dem Gebiete der iusseren Brusper plastik. Leipzig Verlag von Curt Kabitzsch. 1931.
3. Bakamjian VY. A two-stage method for pharyngoesophageal reconstruction with a primary pectoral skin flap. Plast Reconstr Surg. 1965;36(2):173–84. https://doi.org/10.1097/00006534-196508000-00004.
4. Portnoy WM, Arena S. Deltopectoral island flap. Otolaryngol Head Neck Surg. 1994;111(1):63–9. https://doi.org/10.1177/019459989411100113.
5. Stewart CE IV, Urken ML. Deltopectoral flap. In: Fu-Chan Wei SM, editor. Flaps and reconstructive surgery. Elsevier; 2009. p. 193–205.
6. Urken ML. Deltopectoral. In: Atlas of regional and free flaps for head and neck reconstruction. 2nd ed. Lippincott William & Wilkins; 2012. p. 76–88.
7. Daniel RK, Cunningham DM, Taylor IG. The deltopectoral flap: an anatomical and hemodynamic approach. Plast Reconstr Surg. 1975;55(3):275–82.
8. Gingrass RP, Culf NK, Garrett WS, Mladick RA. Complications with the deltopectoral flap. Plast Reconstr Surg. 1972;49(5):501–7. https://doi.org/10.1097/00006534-197205000-00004.
9. Yu P, Roblin P, Chevray P. Internal mammary artery perforator (IMAP) flap for tracheostoma reconstruction. Head Neck. 2006;28:723–9. https://doi.org/10.1002/HED20386.
10. Gilas T, Sako K, Razack MS, Bakamjian VY, Shedd DP, Calamel PM. Major head and neck reconstruction using the deltopectoral flap. A 20 year experience. Am J Surg. 1986;152(4):430–4. https://doi.org/10.1016/0002-9610(86)90318-1.
11. Kass JI, Myers EN. Deltopectoral flap. In: Operative otolaryngology. 3rd ed. Elsevier; 2018. p. 1180–5. https://doi.org/10.1016/B978-0-323-40150-0.00169-7.
12. Mortensen M, Genden EM. Role of the island deltopectoral flap in contemporary head and neck reconstruction. Ann Otol Rhinol Laryngol. 2006;115(5):361–4. https://doi.org/10.1177/000348940611500508.

Facial Artery Myomucosal Flap

3

Daniel P. Russo and Danielle E. Scarola

History

- The facial artery myomucosal (FAMM) flap was first described by Pribatz et al. in 1992 [1].

Indications and Benefits

- Reconstruction of small to moderate sized defects of the hard palate, floor of mouth, upper and lower lip, tongue, alveolus, retromolar trigone, oropharynx, and soft palate [2].
- Pliable, hairless, mucosal flap that is easy to harvest.
- Long length of flap, providing versatility of rotation and coverage.
- Entirety of flap lies deep to muscles of facial expression, thereby protecting the facial nerve.
- The ablative and harvest fields are in immediate proximity to each other with no external scar [3, 4].

Anatomy

- The facial artery branches from the external carotid and courses around the inferior border of the mandible at the antegonial notch anterior to the masseter to enter the face (Fig. 3.1).
- The artery enters the buccal mucosa, 2 cm posterior to the oral commissure.
- Relevant layers with respect to the facial artery in the buccal region are mucosa, submucosa, buccinator muscle, facial artery, terminal branches of the facial nerve, and the muscles of facial expression far laterally.
- The facial artery branches give off the inferior and superior labial artery within the buccal region [5].
- Following the branching of the superior labial artery, the facial artery becomes the angular artery at the level of the nasal ala and terminates at the medial canthus.
- Venous drainage of the harvested flap is from the submucosal venous plexus.
- Stenson's duct limits the total width of the flap, as it lies posteriorly.

D. P. Russo
Division of Otolaryngology- Head and Neck Surgery, Department of Surgery, University of Connecticut School of Medicine, Farmington, CT, USA

D. E. Scarola (✉)
Northwell Health, New York, NY, USA
e-mail: Dscarola@northwell.edu

R. Rezaee, A. Tamaki (eds.), *Local, Regional, and Free Flaps for Head and Neck Reconstruction*,
https://doi.org/10.1007/978-3-032-03211-9_3

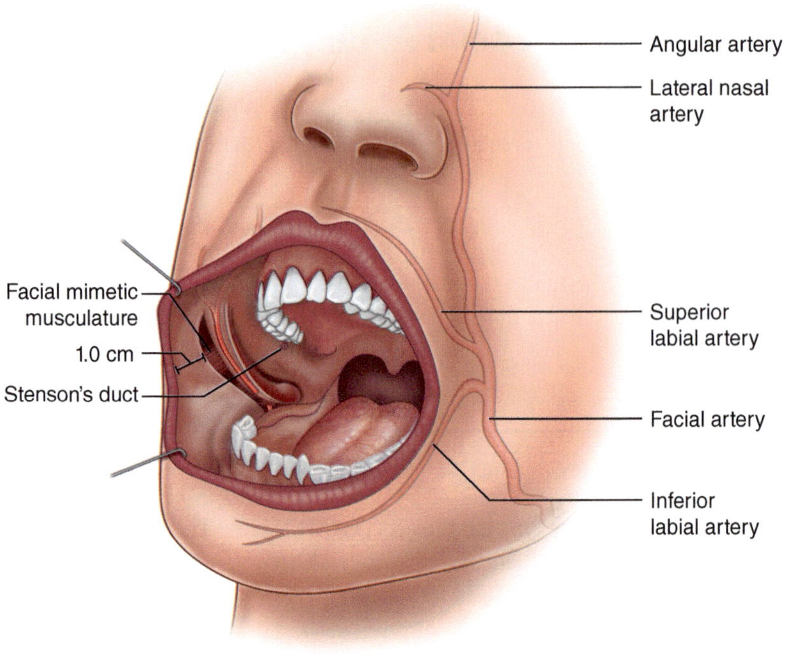

Fig. 3.1 The anatomy of the facial artery myomucosal flap is depicted with its critical arterial, muscular, and soft tissue relationships

Preoperative Care

- Examine the buccal mucosa for cancerous and precancerous lesions in which case the flap should be avoided.
- Ensure patency of facial artery along its course via handheld Doppler.
  - Previous neck dissection with sacrifice of the facial artery makes an inferiorly based flap contraindicated.
  - History of a Caldwell-Luc approach or Weber-Ferguson approach makes a superiorly based flap contraindicated.
- History of oral cavity radiation is a relative contraindication as it increases risk of complications and reduces the size and pliability of the flap. Therefore, it should be used with caution in these patients.
- Preoperative antibiotic prophylaxis directed against oral cavity flora should be considered.

Special Instruments and Positioning

- Weider cheek and tongue retractor.
- Gillies skin hooks, traction sutures, or self-retaining cheek retractors for upper and lower lip retraction.
- Handheld Doppler is helpful to trace the vascular pedicle.
- Position the endotracheal tube (ETT) contralateral to the surgical bed.
- Securing ETT to the dentition contralateral to harvest site with suture or wire can improve retraction of cheek and lips limited by standard ETT taping.
- Neuromuscular blockade (to ease mouth opening) is recommended [5].

Modifications

- The pedicle can be based superiorly or inferiorly, depending on the defect [6].
- While FAMM flap often requires a second-stage procedure to divide the bridging pedicle over the dentition or alveolus, a single-staged approach has been described.
- An island FAMM flap involves transecting the mucosa at the base and leaving the flap pedicled solely on the facial artery and adjacent tissue. This relies on the venae comitantes within the soft tissue surrounding the artery for venous return [7].

Pitfalls and Complications

- Given the uncertainty of primary resection in many cases, surgeons must consent the patient for alternative reconstructive options, which may include a microvascular free flap or other regional flaps.
- Involvement of level I of the neck could result in facial artery sacrifice, making an inferiorly based flap contraindicated. If a two-team approach is planned, preoperative and post-ablative communication between the ablative team and reconstructive team about the status of the facial artery is advised.
- Local infiltration of epinephrine into the surgical bed can result in spasm of the facial artery and complicate dissection and, therefore, is not recommended.
- If a smaller flap width is desired, the posterior incision can be moved more anteriorly, away from Stenson's duct. However, anteriorly, 1 cm from the oral commissure must be maintained (facial artery can traverse near the anterior margin) [2].
- Partial necrosis is the most common complication with tip necrosis being more common than base necrosis.
- Surgical site infections.
- Infrequently cheek hematoma, tongue tethering, and trismus have been described [4, 5].

Postoperative Care

- Pedicle of the flap will cross from the alveolar crest over the gingiva, often requiring a second stage for division of the pedicle at least 3 weeks after initial surgery.
  - Second-stage procedure may be indicated if bulk from the pedicle interferes with dental rehabilitation, mobility of the tongue, or mouth closure.
- If the pedicle crosses intact dentition, a bite-block should be placed for approximately 10 days to protect the pedicle. This can be from a variety of materials prefabricated or created from rolled gauze.
- No drain placement required [2].

Tissue Type: *Myomucosal*
Artery: *Facial artery*
Vein: *Submucosal venous plexus*
Nerve: *None*
Flap reach: *Can extend up to 9 cm to reach defects of the oral cavity and oropharynx*
Flap size: *Maximum 8–9 cm in length × 3 cm in width*

Operative Procedure

Inferiorly-Based FAMM Flap

1. Design the flap on the buccal mucosa according to the following borders:
   - Anterior: 1 cm posterior to the oral commissure.
   - Posterior: Limited by the Stenson's duct.
   - Inferior: Base should be 2–3 cm wide and centered over second molar.
   - Superior: Extends to the gingivolabial sulcus.
2. Locate the facial artery through distal (posterior) or proximal (anterior) identification. Doppler can be useful for identification and design of the flap.
   - *Distal identification*: Incise the mucosa, submucosa, and buccinator muscle at the distal edge of the flap. Identify the facial artery deep to the buccinator and clip distally.

- *Proximal identification*: Initiate dissection 1 cm lateral to the oral commissure through the mucosa, submucosa, and buccinator muscle. Identify the superior labial artery. Follow the superior labial artery proximally to its origin off the facial artery. Clip the superior labial artery and proceed with dissection.

3. Elevate the flap in the plane just deep to the facial artery, including the buccinator muscle.
4. Inset the flap by rotating it inferiorly and closing it with horizontal mattress sutures.
5. Close the donor site with interrupted horizontal mattress sutures [1, 2, 5]. Gentle blunt dissection and removal of any retraction devices can assist with closure.

Superiorly-Based FAMM Flap

The operative technique is largely similar aside from several key alterations described as follows:

1. Design the flap with the pivot point in the gingivolabial sulcus at the first molar.
   * Preserve 0.5–1.0 cm between the gingiva and the posterior margin.
2. Locate the facial artery through either anterior (proximal) identification (as above) or posterior (distal) identification (Fig. 3.1).
   - *Anterior identification*: Incise past the buccinator at the inferior (distal) margin of the flap, identify the facial artery, and clip.
3. Elevate the flap from distal to proximal relative to the flap, in a plane just deep to the facial artery.
   * The superior course of the facial artery is tortuous, requiring meticulous dissection [6].

Single-Staged Procedure

The operative technique for a single-staged procedure involves extending the anterior incision across the alveolar ridge to meet with the posterior aspect of the floor of mouth defect.

1. Along the alveolar ridge, incision is carried submucosally or subperiosteally to free the base and allow rotation. This allows the anterior edge of the flap to be closed to the medial aspect of the defect.
2. Alternatively, a mucosal island can be created by transecting the flap's mucosa at its base while leaving the artery and immediate adjacent tissue intact as noted above [7].

Disclosure Statement No conflicts of interest to disclose.

References

1. Pribaz J, Stephens W, Crespo L, Gifford G. A new intraoral flap. Plast Reconstr Surg. 1992;90:421–9.
2. Ayad T. Facial artery musculomucosal (FAMM) flap. Oper Tech Otolaryngol Head Neck Surg. 2019;30:112–9.
3. Massarelli O, Vaira LA, De Riu G. Islanded facial artery musculomucosal flap for tongue reconstruction. Int J Oral Max Surg. 2015;46:1060–1.
4. Ayad T, Kolb F, Monés ED, Mamelle G, Temam S. Reconstruction of floor of mouth defects by the facial artery musculo-mucosal flap following cancer ablation. Head Neck. 2008;30:437–45.
5. Ayad T, Xie L. Facial artery musculomucosal flap in head and neck reconstruction: a systematic review. Head Neck. 2015;37:1375–86.
6. Berania I, Lavigne F, Rahal A, Ayad T. Superiorly based facial artery musculomucosal flap: a versatile pedicled flap. Head Neck. 2018;40:402–5.
7. Duranceau M, Ayad T. The facial artery musculomucosal flap: modification of the harvesting technique for a single-stage procedure. Laryngoscope. 2011;121:2586–9.

4 Infraclavicular Pedicled Adipofascial Flap

Akshay V. Patel

History

- First introduced in the literature as a fasciocutaneous free flap by Yoo and Belzile in 2014 [1].
- The pedicled adipofascial infraclavicular flap was described in 2016 [2].
- Alain et al. modified the pedicle flap to include fasciocutaneous tissue [3].

Indications and Benefits

- Uses of the pedicled adipofascial flap include:
  - Vascular coverage.
  - Contouring the neck after radical neck dissection and loss of sternocleidomastoid muscle.
  - Skin graft recipient bed in the setting of an open neck defect.
  - Vascularized onlay following pharyngeal closure.
  - Obliteration of cervical dead space.
  - Coverage of cervical spine hardware.
- Uses of the pedicled fasciocutaneous flap include:
  - Augmentation of pharyngeal lumen.
  - Cutaneous defect reconstruction inferior to the mandible.
- The flap can be raised quickly (15–30 min) with minimal blood loss.
- The flap is reliable and well vascularized.
- Visual identification of a vascular pedicle is not required.
- Harvest of the flap still preserves the pectoralis major myofascial flap.

Anatomy

- The infraclavicular adipofascial flap is vascularized by the anterior perforator of the transverse cervical artery (Fig. 4.1) [1, 4].
  - The anterior perforator of the transverse cervical artery runs over the posterior belly of the omohyoid muscle in the anteroinferior direction and superficial to the clavicle.
  - The anterior perforator runs between the platysma and the deltopectoral fascia.
- The venous drainage is through the external jugular vein and less commonly the transverse cervical vein.

A. V. Patel (✉)
Connecticut Institute of Head and Neck Surgery, Hartford, CT, USA

Hartford HealthCare Cancer Institute, Hartford, CT, USA

Hartford Hospital Department of Otolaryngology-Head and Neck Surgery, Hartford, CT, USA
Apatel@ctentonline.com

R. Rezaee, A. Tamaki (eds.), *Local, Regional, and Free Flaps for Head and Neck Reconstruction*,
https://doi.org/10.1007/978-3-032-03211-9_4

Preoperative Care

- It is important to identify if a patient has had previous disruption to the transverse cervical artery and proximal external jugular vein from prior neck surgery.
- Preservation of the transverse cervical artery, proximal external jugular vein, and omohyoid muscle during the ablation are essential.
- Assess for history or scars from prior surgery or trauma that may compromise vascular anatomy or perfusion to the skin (e.g., pacemaker, breast implant, implanted port).

Special Instruments and Positioning

- Doppler may aid in identification of the anterior perforator of the transverse cervical artery.

Modifications

- Can be harvested as a fasciocutaneous flap.
- Can be harvested as a free flap.
  - When used as a free flap the pedicle length is variable. Artery can be lengthened by de-epithelializing the proximal skin component and dissecting to the thyrocervical trunk.
  - The vein can be lengthened by using the external jugular vein in retrograde fashion (this may require valvulectomy) [1].

Pitfalls and Complications

- Inadvertent subplatysmal plane harvesting risking injury to the anterior perforator of the transverse cervical artery.
- Elevating an overlying skin flap that is too thin resulting in skin necrosis, particularly in a radiated patient.
- Seroma formation, particularly in adipose-rich patients.

Postoperative Care

- Dress the incision with a bandage for 2 days.
- Maintain a closed suction drain for 5–7 days or even longer among adipose-rich patients.
- Initiate arm range of motion exercises immediately.

Tissue type: *Adipofascial, fasciocutaneous*
Artery: *Anterior perforator of the transverse cervical artery*
Vein: *External jugular vein, transverse cervical vein*
Flap reach: *Can cover the ipsilateral neck to the inferior aspect of the mandible*
Flap size: *Adipofascial flap: 25 × 25 cm; fasciocutaneous flap: 10 × 7 cm*

Operative Procedure

1. Mark the ipsilateral clavicle and fashion an 8–10 cm transverse skin marking parallel and two fingerbreadths caudad to the inferior border of the clavicle.
2. Using a Doppler, identify and mark the signal of the anterior perforator of the transverse cervical artery. This is usually found at the junction between the lateral two-thirds and medial one-third of the clavicle (Fig. 4.1).
3. A line can be drawn from the Doppler point to the anterior axillary line to isolate the course of the anterior perforator.
4. Sharply make an incision through the skin and immediate subcutaneous tissue.
5. Identify the platysma, but do not divide it as this is the superficial aspect of the flap.

   * Among thin and elderly patients, the platysma can be difficult to identify in the infraclavicular region, but it can be traced or approximated from the neck.

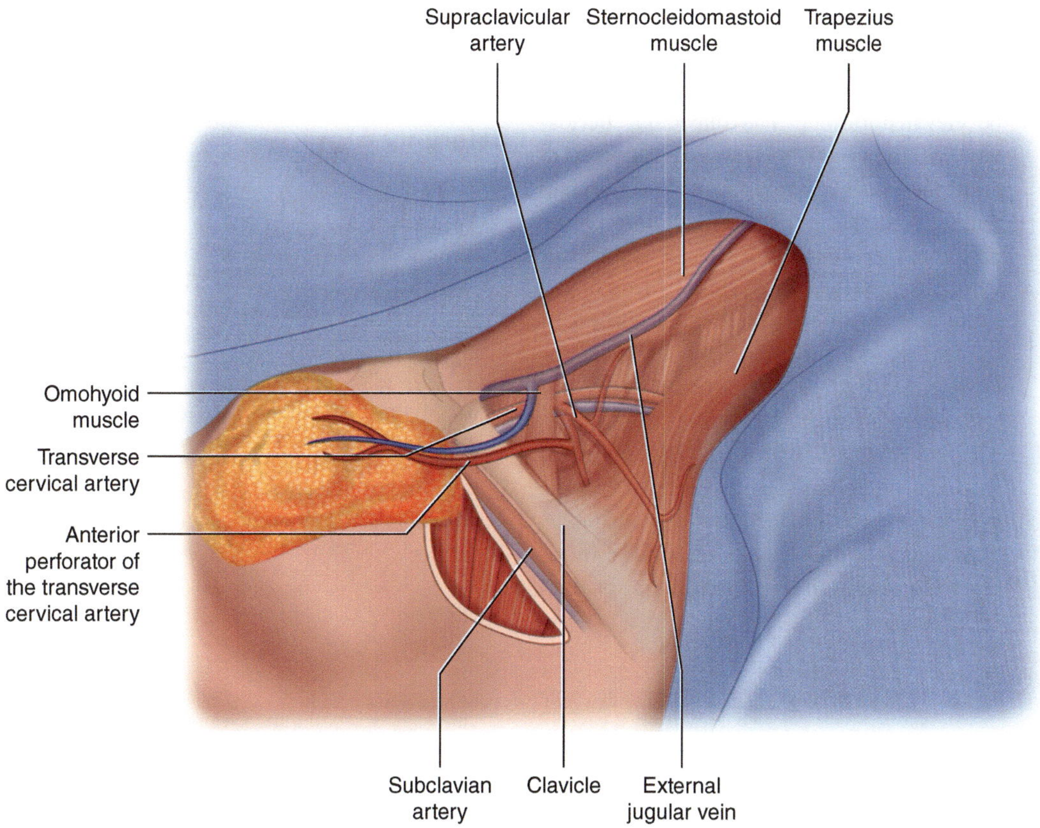

Fig. 4.1 The infraclavicular adipofascial flap is depicted with its blood supply from the anterior perforator of the transverse cervical artery. Venous drainage is often through the external jugular vein

6. Raise a superior supraplatysmal flap transitioning to the subplatysmal plane in the neck above the level of the omohyoid at a level to not disrupt the course of the anterior perforator as it courses over the omohyoid and under the inferior most aspect of the platysma as the vessel crosses the clavicle. This dissection will help create a wide tunnel through which the flap will be transposed superiorly into the neck defect.
7. Raise an inferior supraplatysmal skin flap to the desired inferior extent of flap harvest.
8. With the skin flaps retracted, divide through the underlying adipofascial tissue and through the pectoralis major fascia (but not the pectoralis major muscle) medially, inferiorly, and laterally to the desired flap size.
9. Grasp the inferior aspect of the flap with two to three atraumatic clamps and retrograde dissect the flap to elevate it toward the clavicle in a subfascial plane along the surface of the pectoralis major muscle.
10. As the clavicle is approached the flap can be flipped into the neck through the created tunnel so that the superficial surface is now deep.

* If additional length is needed, the periosteum of the clavicle can be incised to protect the anterior perforator and the flap can be elevated further. The clavicular periosteum can be carefully elevated superiorly to allow for further mobilization of the flap without concern for damaging the perforator.

11. Check for perfusion by sharply excising a small amount of the distal most portion of the flap to assess for bleeding and/or identifying the signal of the anterior perforator with a sterile handheld Doppler.
12. The flap is secured with absorbable suture to the local tissue based on position, coverage needs, and area planned for contouring. A closed suction drain is placed and the infraclavicular incision is closed in a layered fashion.

Disclosure Statement No conflicts of interest to disclose.

References

1. Yoo J, Belzile M. Infraclavicular free flap for head and neck reconstruction: surgical description and early outcomes in 7 consecutive patients. Head Neck. 2015;37:309–16. https://doi.org/10.1002/hed.23597.
2. Yoo J, Low TH, Tam S, Partridge A, MacNeil D, Nichols A, Fung K. Head Neck. 2016;38:1579–82. https://doi.org/10.1002/hed.24472.
3. Alain C, Fortier PH, Belzile M. The infraclavicular pedicled flap in head and neck reconstruction: applications and outcomes. Head Neck. 2020;42:77–84. https://doi.org/10.1002/hed.25990.
4. Pallua N, Wolter TP. Moving forwards: the anterior supraclavicular artery perforator (a-SAP) flap. J Plast Reconstr Aesthet Surg. 2013;66:489–96.

5 Lower Trapezius Myocutaneous Flap

Matthew Old, Robert Sinard, and James Netterville

History

- The lower trapezius myocutaneous flap was first described by Baek et al. in 1980, 1 year after the description of the pectoralis flap [1].
- The pectoralis flap, with its ease of harvest, overshadowed the trapezius flap and became the workhorse of head and neck reconstruction. The lower trapezius flap requires more difficult patient positioning and does not have the extended utility of the pectoralis flap for oral cavity and pharyngeal reconstruction. However, for lateral and posterior skull defects, it is far superior to the pectoralis flap or other regional flaps.

Indications and Benefits

- Reconstruction of large defects on the lateral or posterior surface of the head and neck and potential use for oral cavity and oropharyngeal defects.
- Reliable reconstructive option in patients where the free flap is not an option.
- Thin and pliable tissue with excellent arc of rotation.
- Well-camouflaged donor incision on the back.
- Can be harvested with no deficits to shoulder elevation and function as the upper trapezius muscle fibers along with the spinal accessory nerve are preserved [2].

Anatomy

- Trapezius muscle is a thin and broad triangular muscle that covers the posterior neck and upper back.
  - Muscle attaches to superior nuchal line, external occipital protuberance, nuchal ligament, and spinous processes of the seventh cervical to 12th thoracic vertebrae.
- In the initial description of the flap, the transverse cervical artery (TCA) was described as the major blood supply to this lower trapezius region but found that this led to poor vascularity of the distal portion of the flap [1].

M. Old (✉)
Department of Otolaryngology- Head and Neck Surgery, University of Washington Medicine, Seattle, WA, USA

R. Sinard · J. Netterville
Department of Otolaryngology- Head and Neck Surgery, Vanderbilt University Medical Center, Nashville, TN, USA
e-mail: Robert.Sinard@Vanderbilt.edu

R. Rezaee, A. Tamaki (eds.), *Local, Regional, and Free Flaps for Head and Neck Reconstruction*,
https://doi.org/10.1007/978-3-032-03211-9_5

- After careful review of the anatomy of the trapezius vasculature, the dorsal scapular artery (DSA) was found to provide the major portion of the blood supply to the fibers of the trapezius muscle and its overlying skin inferior to the scapular spine [3].
- Skin overlying the trapezius muscle receives its blood supply from four sources: TCA, DSA, intercostal artery, and occipital artery [3, 4].
  - TCA and DSA contribute blood supply to cutaneous regions overlying the trapezius muscle such that a myocutaneous flap can be elevated based on either or both arteries.
  - However, the DSA provides a far more robust supply to the lower portion of the flap providing for a much longer pedicle to transfer.
- TCA originates from the thyrocervical trunk. It then passes over the brachial plexus and the levator muscle before descending in the investing fascia on the deep surface of the superior trapezius muscle (Figs. 5.1 and 5.2).
- DSA takes its origin from the subclavian artery just lateral to the anterior scalene insertion.
  - This branch is approximately 2 cm lateral to the origin of the thyrocervical trunk.
  - The DSA then travels between the branches of the brachial plexus and takes a very serpentine course as it dives under the levator muscle deep to the superior angle of the scapula (Fig. 5.1). It divides at the level of the scapular spine.
  - The major branch penetrates between the rhomboid major and minor muscles, then descends along the deep surface of the trapezius to supply the inferior trapezius region (Fig. 5.2).
  - Smaller branch, or branches, travel deep to the rhomboid major, yielding several small muscular perforators that may pass laterally through the rhomboid major into the trapezius in a more inferior position (Fig. 5.3).
- Cadaver dissection explored the clinical variations of these two arteries [3].
  - In most of the dissections, either the DSA or the TCA was usually the dominant vessel. The dominant vessel was larger than the nondominant vessel and, the proximal portion of the nondominant vessel often did not

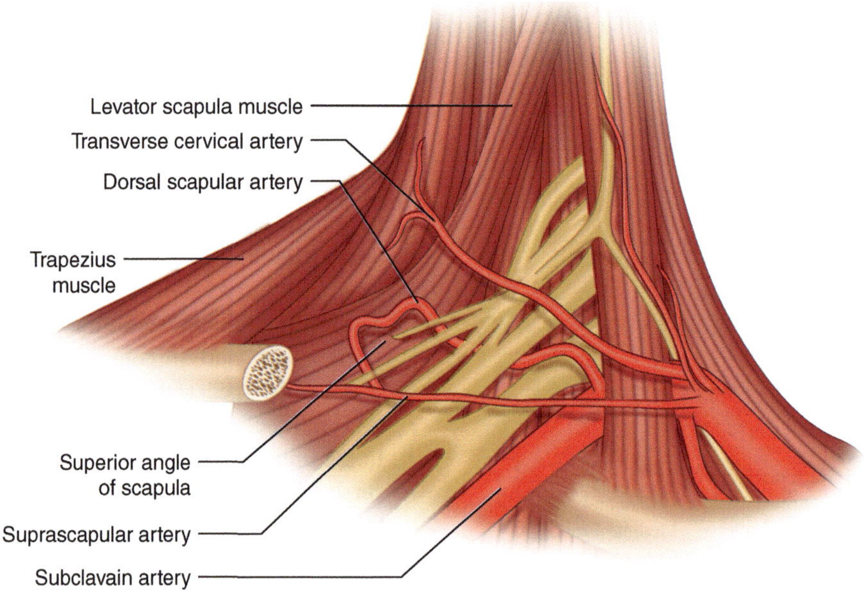

Fig. 5.1 This diagram demonstrates the more commonly described course of the transverse cervical artery over the levator muscle, and the dorsal scapular artery, passing through the brachial plexus, then diving deep to the levator muscle

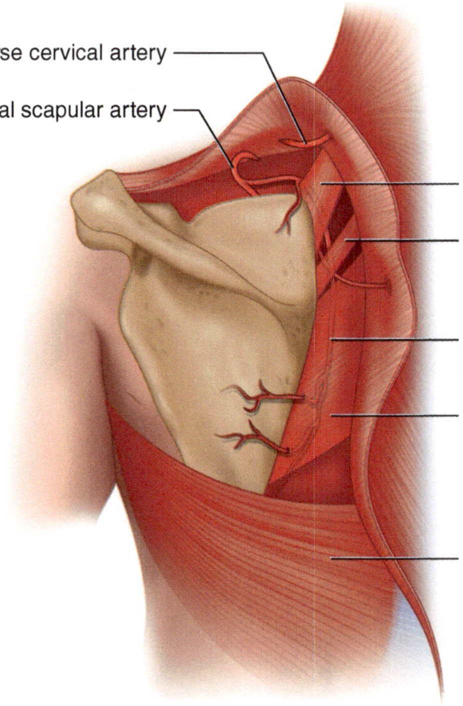

Fig. 5.2 The distal portion of the dorsal scapular artery traverses deep to the levator and the scapula, then divides at the level of the scapular spine. The major branch passes below the lower edges of the rhomboid minor and above the upper border of the rhomboid major. The major portion of the artery passes in the deep fascia of the trapezius muscle sending small branches into the muscle. It also sends a small branch deep the rhomboid major that must be ligated

exist or was less than 1 mm in diameter with no distal connection to the trapezius. This resulted in variations in the proximal arterial anatomy, but the vascular anatomy distal to the levator muscle was always consistent, with the TCA following its usual pattern over the levator muscle and the DSA traveling in its usual path deep to the levator muscle and the upper border of the scapula.

- When a proximal dominant artery occurred, then the distal portion of both the DSA and the TCA arose from that dominant vessel.
  - When the TCA was dominant, the DSA branched off of it just proximal to the levator muscle and passed deep to it in its usual and customary course (Fig. 5.4).
  - When the DSA was the dominant vessel, the TCA branched off of it just proximal to the levator and passed over the levator in its usual and customary course (Fig. 5.5).
- The proximal diameter of the vessels when dominant averaged 2.25 mm for the TCA and 2.75 mm for the DSA.
- The average size of the distal portion of the DSA, as it penetrated the trapezius muscle just medial to the scapular spine, was 1.75 mm.
- The ink injection studies in fresh cadavers demonstrated ink distribution in the cutaneous segment that could be predicted based on the dominance of the vessel injected. In dissections with vessels of equal caliber, injection of the TCA caused ink staining of the skin above the level of the rhomboid minor while injection of the DSA showed most of the cutaneous staining below the level of the rhomboid minor with some staining above, demonstrating a much broader blood supply for dependable harvest of the lower positioned flap.

• Venous drainage is from the transverse cervical vein (TCV), which may be a single or dual vein that exits the trapezius muscle on its deep surface [5].
• Motor innervation to the trapezius muscle includes cranial nerve XI, while sensory innervation is supplied though the second to fourth cervical nerves.

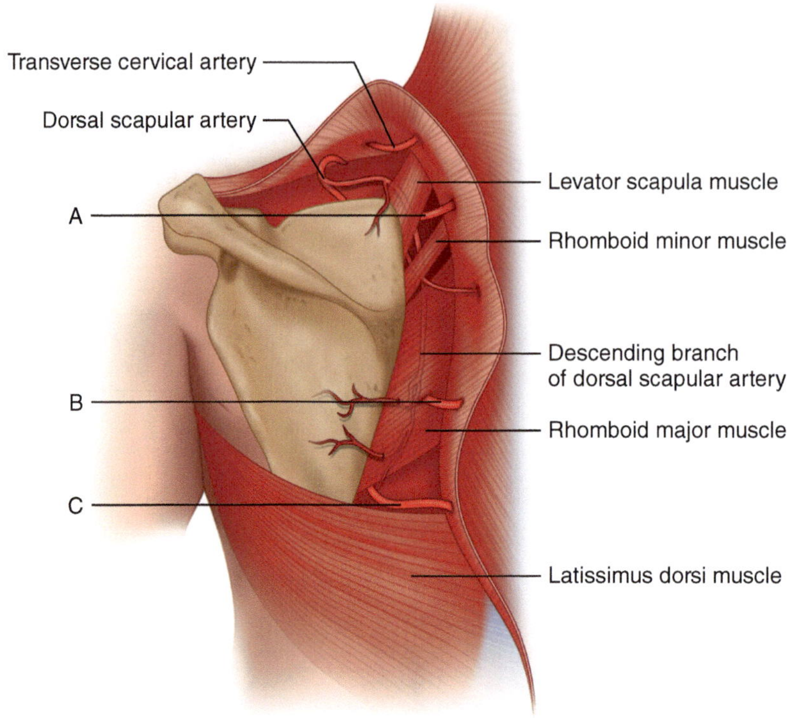

Fig. 5.3 This figure demonstrates the variations of the dorsal scapular artery as it enters the trapezius muscle. Very rarely the artery sends a substantial branch into the muscle superior the rhomboid minor muscle (**a**). This branch will normally be automatically incorporated into the flap. Descending off the major branch of the dorsal scapular that enters the muscle just below the rhomboid minor are two variations of less important branches that can be ligated as needed. This descending branch can penetrate through the mid portion of the rhomboid major (**b**) and enter the lower trapezius or it can pass inferior the rhomboid major and enter into the inferior trapezius

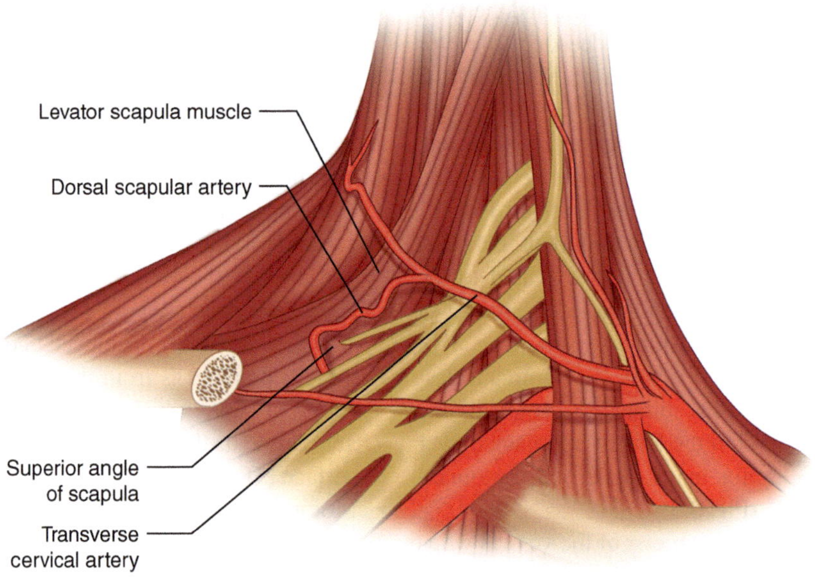

Fig. 5.4 This diagram depicts the less common vascular variation showing the dorsal scapular artery arising from the dominant transverse cervical artery, then passing in its normal course deep to the levator muscle

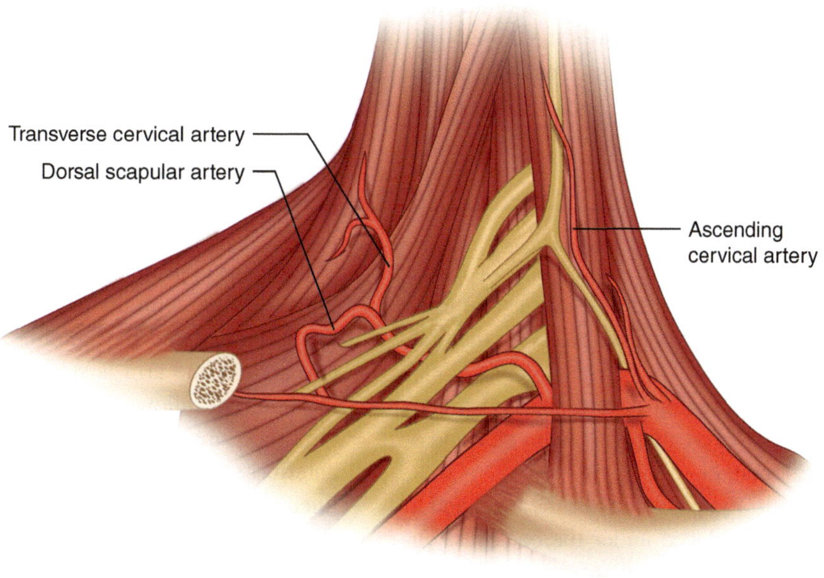

Fig. 5.5 This diagram depicts the more common vascular variation, with the transverse cervical artery arising from the dominant dorsal scapular artery and passing in its normal course over the levator muscle

Preoperative Care

- Caution must be used in patient with previous ipsilateral neck dissection.
  - If the TCA has been sacrificed in that dissection, contrasted imaging should be performed to examine the vascular anatomy to ensure the DSA is intact and providing the major blood supply to the lower trapezius region.

Special Instruments and Positioning

- Patient is positioned in the lateral decubitus (or prone) position depending on defect location, then prepped and draped so that the back is visible down to the iliac crest and past the midline as identified by the spinous processes.
- Ipsilateral area of the arm is kept free of arterial or venous access lines and is sterilely draped into the field. This allows for its mobility during the procedure.
- Positioning in the lateral decubitus position allows for a two-team approach and prevents an intraoperative change of position, which always risks breaks in surgical techniques and sterility.

Modifications

- Trapezius system regional flaps consist of three distinct flaps, one of which is the lateral trapezius myocutaneous flaps. The additional two are the superior trapezius flap and the lateral island trapezius flap.
- There is potential for harvesting bone (including the scapula), which can be incorporated into the flap.

Pitfalls and Complications

- Patient must be positioned in the lateral decubitus (or prone) position, but two team approach is possible.
- It is important for the harvesting surgeon to understand the vascular variations to this flap to ensure greater success. The distal anatomy of the two arteries are constant; however, the proximal

blood supply to the cutaneous region of the flap can arise from either the TCA or the DSA.
- Possibility of distal flap loss, especially when extended beyond the lower border of the muscle [5].

Postoperative Care

- The area of rotation of the DSA must be protected from pressure on the vessels for the first 10 days.
- The vulnerable region is outlined and a "no pressure sign" is created with foam tape and a permanent marker.
- A small pillow is placed under the head and a large pillow is placed under the back just on the side of the dissection inferior to the "no pressure sign." This is usually very comfortable for the patient. While the patient is in the bed, these pillows are maintained until postoperative day 10.

Tissue type: *Myocutaneaus, myogenous*
Artery: *Dorsal scapular artery with contributions from the transverse cervical, intercostal, and occipital artery*
Vein: *Transverse cervical vein*
Nerve: *Cranial nerve XI, second to fourth cervical nerve*
Flap reach: *Reported reach to midface, oral cavity, and oropharynx*
Flap size: *Lower extent of flap up to 15 cm below the inferior border of the scapula*

Operative Procedure

1. The patient is positioned in the lateral decubitus position, with the back visible down to the iliac crest and past midline. The ipsilateral area of the arm is sterilely draped into the field and allows for its mobility during the procedure. After the arm is placed in an anteriorly rotated position, the flap is outlined over the lower medial trapezius fibers (Fig. 5.6). Arm holding devices can be considered to aid with positioning based on body habitus.
2. The medial edge of the flap is placed as close to the midline as possible, which allows a greater distal extension of the flap still overlying the inferior aspect of the trapezius muscle.

   * The flap is purposely outlined too long and later tailored to fit the size of the surgical defect. This increase in paddle length allows for more cosmetic closure of the back incision with less dog-ear formation at each end, as well as allowing for the inclusion of more

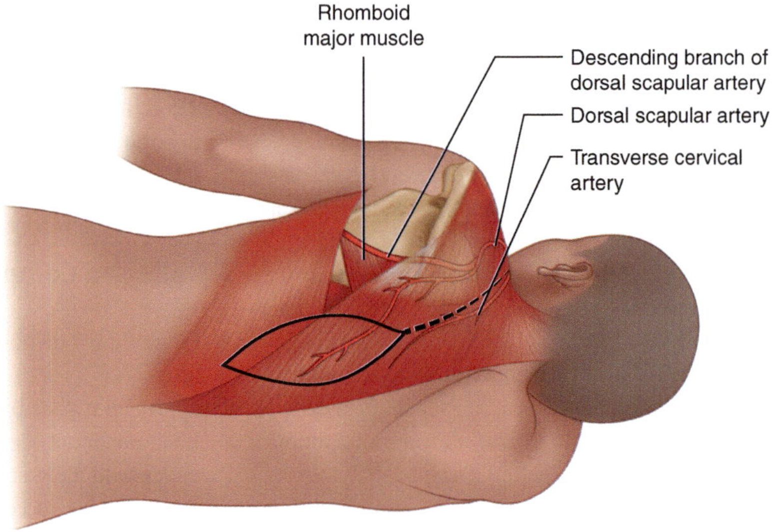

Fig. 5.6 The lateral decubitus position allows for primary resection of ipsilateral head and neck lesions as well as for harvest of the trapezius flap with no intraoperative change

potential perforators into the subcutaneous aspect of the flap.

* The distal aspect of the flap may extend 15 cm below the tip of the scapula, which creates a significant random extension on the inferior lateral aspect of the skin paddle.

3. The outlined skin paddle is incised and elevated over the latissimus dorsi muscle starting on the inferior lateral border. Following this plane medially, identify the lower trapezius muscle fibers.
4. The flap is further elevated deep to the trapezius until the lower border of the rhomboid major is identified.

   * In most situations, this muscle is left in place, which prevents postoperative winging of the scapula.
5. At this point, the distal arcade of the dorsal scapular artery is usually identified in the deep fascia on the undersurface of the trapezius muscle. It is followed up until it departs from the muscle at the interface between the rhomboid minor and the rhomboid major muscles adjacent to the medial portion of the scapular spine (Fig. 5.7).
6. In most cases, additional pedicle length is needed at this point. The descending branches of the DSA that pass deep to the rhomboid major are ligated and divided.

   * In 20% of the cases, there are two or three sets of descending vessels that must be divided. After this division, gentle dissection along the DSA allows one to uncoil it from its serpentine path under the scapula.

   * This allows for an additional 2–3 cm of pedicle length.

   * If further rotation is needed, the rhomboid minor is divided on either side of the vascular pedicle, which allows for several more centimeters of rotation with no venous tension (Fig. 5.8).

   * If necessary, one may cut the DSA and continue the superior muscle division allowing the flap to be vascularized only by the more superiorly positioned TCA. This works well for flaps positioned above the level of the scapula tip, but skin paddles positioned inferior to the scapula tip may suffer from arterial insufficiency without input from the DSA.
7. The upper trapezius fibers are divided superiorly just enough to rotate the distal portion of the skin paddle into the defect, protecting the superior portion of the muscle.

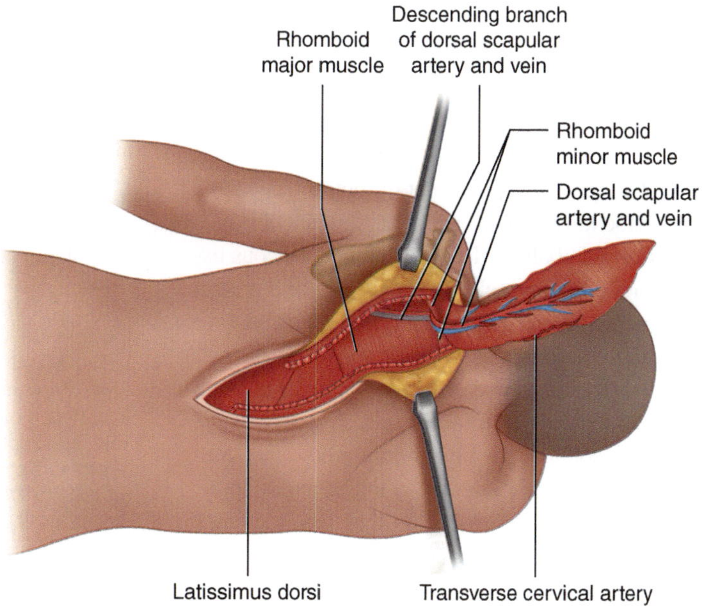

Fig. 5.7 The major branch of the dorsal scapular artery is identified just medial to the scapular spine passing between the rhomboid major and the rhomboid minor muscles

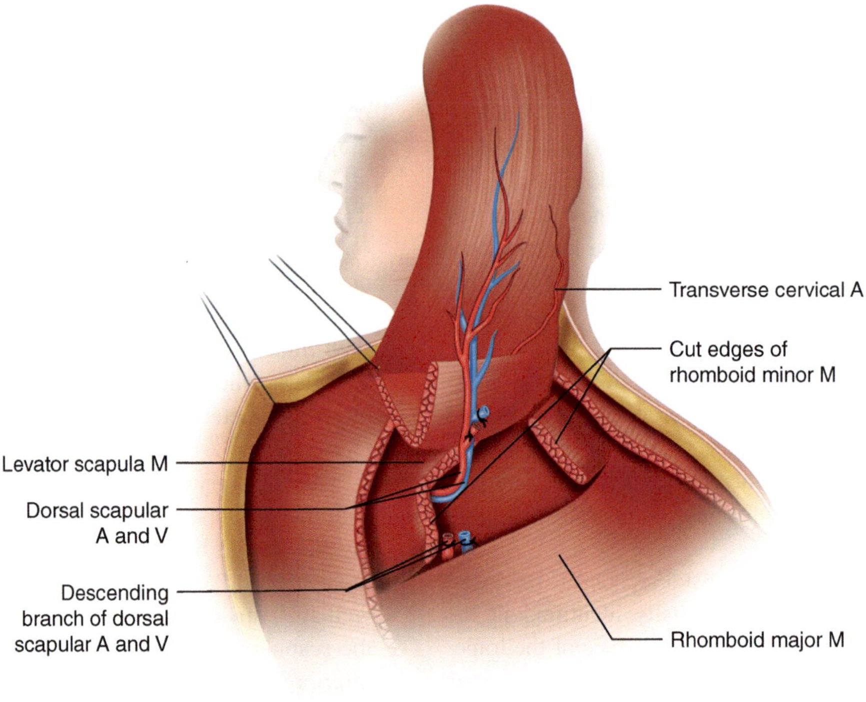

Fig. 5.8 To extend the pedicle length of the flap. The descending branch of the dorsal scapular artery is divided, and the rhomboid minor muscle is either partially or totally divided both from its medial and lateral attachments. This allows the deep portion of the dorsal scapular artery to uncoil, adding length to the pedicle

* This allows for normal shoulder elevation postoperatively.

8. The flap can then be either passed through a subcutaneous tunnel or (the safer) complete incision up to the defect to be placed into a pharyngeal defect or (more commonly) rotated onto a temporo-cutaneous (or posterior) defect (Fig. 5.8).
9. If the proximal portion of the cutaneous paddle is too long, then the necessary amount of skin is de-epithelialized, leaving the subcutaneous tissues on the muscle, thus allowing for a greater subcutaneous muscle interface, which ensures more perforators into the cutaneous tissue.
10. The back is closed primarily with care taken to avoid pressure on the vessels. Postoperatively, the patient is positioned on a pillow that contacts the back inferior to the scapular spine. This prevents pressure on the vessels as they rotate over the superior trapezius fibers.

Disclosure Statement No conflicts of interest to disclose.

References

1. Baek SM, Biller HF, Krespi YP, Lawson W. The lower trapezius Island myocutaneous flap. Ann Plast Surg. 1980;5(2):108–14. https://doi.org/10.1097/00000637-198008000-00004.
2. Mathes SJ, Nahai F. Muscle flap transposition with function preservation: technical and clinical considerations. Plast Reconstr Surg. 1980;66(2):242–9. https://doi.org/10.1097/00006534-198008000-00013.
3. Netterville JL, Wood DE. The lower trapezius flap. Vascular anatomy and surgical technique. Arch Otolaryngol Head Neck Surg. 1991;117(1):73–6. https://doi.org/10.1001/archotol.1991.01870130079020.
4. Urken ML, Naidu RK, Lawson W, Biller HF. The lower trapezius Island musculocutaneous flap revisited. Report of 45 cases and a unifying concept of the vascular supply. Arch Otolaryngol Head Neck Surg. 1991;117(5):502–11. https://doi.org/10.1001/archotol.1991.01870170048012.
5. Goodwin WJ, Rosenberg GJ. Venous drainage of the lateral trapezius musculocutaneous Island flap. Arch Otolaryngol. 1982;108(7):411–3. https://doi.org/10.1001/archotol.1982.00790550015004.

6 Melolabial Flap

Mingyang L. Gray and Marita S. Teng

History

- First described in 600 BC in the Hindu works of Sushruta as a local flap from the lower part of the cheek to reconstruct the nose [1].
- Resurfaced in the mid-1800s in Europe for repair of nasal alar defects and popularized again after World War II.
- The terms melolabial and nasolabial flap are often used interchangeably, but melolabial may be more accurate, given the flap tissue is located along the crease separating the cheek (prefix melo-) from the lip (suffix -labial).

Indications and Benefits

- Reconstruction of the nose.
  - Lower third (alar, nasal tip, columella) and middle third (nasal sidewall).
  - Excellent color match for the lower third of the nose.
- Reconstruction of the oral cavity (e.g., buccal, palatal, tongue, alveolus, lip, and floor of mouth).
- Reconstruction of various facial defects (e.g., cheek, lower eyelid, and chin).
- Robust vascularity with low failure rate [2].
- Versatile and can be used as a one-stage transposition flap or two-stage interpolated flap.
- Donor scar hides in melolabial crease.

Anatomy

- The melolabial crease separates the cheek from the lips and runs obliquely from 1 cm superior to the lateral alar rim to 1 cm lateral to the corner of the mouth (Fig. 6.1) [3].
- Skin from the medial canthus of the eye to the inferior margin of the mandible can be incorporated into the melolabial flap.
- The melolabial flap can be harvested as a random or axial pattern flap.
- Blood supply is from the facial (including its terminal branch, the angular artery), infraorbital, and transverse facial artery [4–6].
- Venous drainage is based on the subdermal plexus, including the facial vein.
- Muscles of facial expression present in this region including the risorius, levator labii superioris, levator labii superioris alaeque nasi, and zygomatic major and minor muscles [3].
  - The facial artery typically runs deep to these muscles and superficial to the buccinator and levator anguli oris muscles, but this relationship can vary.

M. L. Gray (✉) · M. S. Teng
Department of Otolaryngology- Head and Neck Surgery, Icahn School of Medicine at Mount Sinai, New York, NY, USA
e-mail: marita.teng@mountsinai.org

R. Rezaee, A. Tamaki (eds.), *Local, Regional, and Free Flaps for Head and Neck Reconstruction*,
https://doi.org/10.1007/978-3-032-03211-9_6

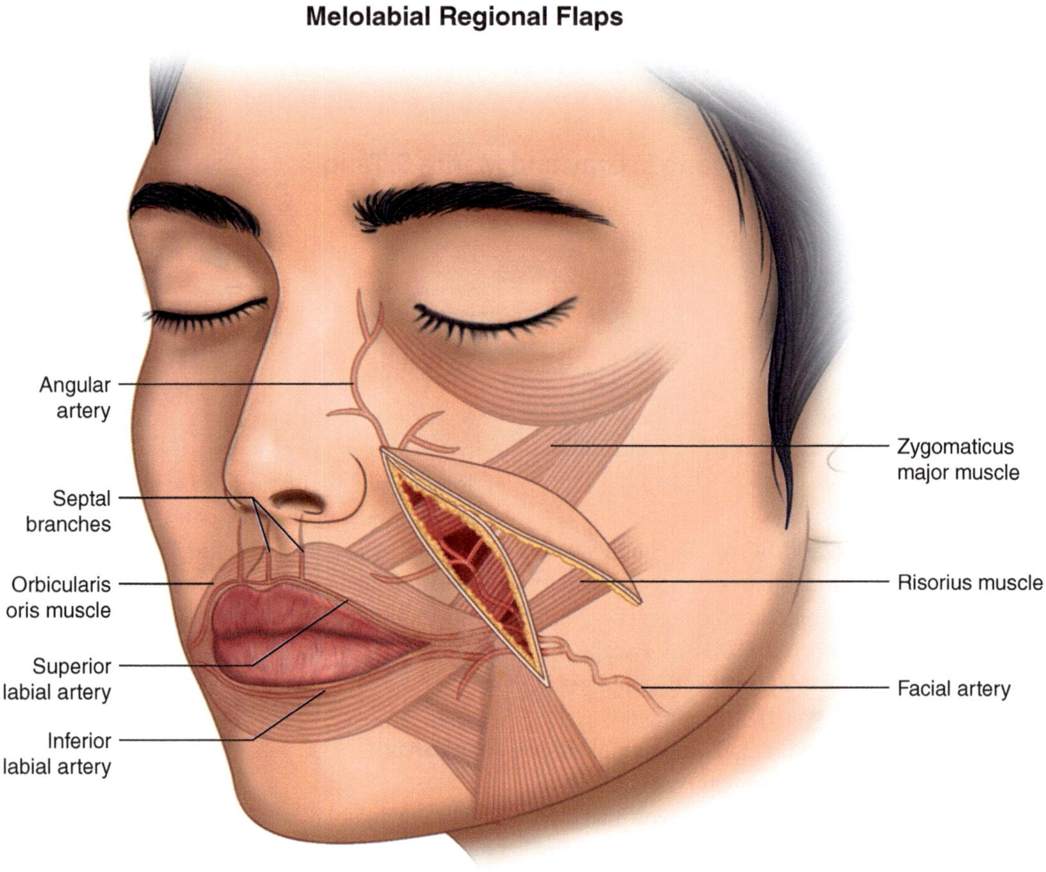

Fig. 6.1 The melolabial flap is a random or axial pattern flap supplied primarily by the facial artery. Flaps can be designed with an inferiorly, superiorly, or centrally based pedicles (superiorly depicted here). Branches of the facial artery and muscles of facial expression in the region are shown

- Superficial musculoaponeurotic system (SMAS) surrounds the facial mimetic muscles, which send fibrous attachments to the dermal layer of the skin at the level of the melolabial fold [4].
- Thickness can vary, with significant subcutaneous fat lateral to the melolabial crease but minimal fat overlying the orbicularis oris medial to the crease.
- The buccal and zygomatic branches of the facial nerve innervate the majority of the muscles of facial expression from the deep aspect [3].

Preoperative Care

- Managing patient expectations and counseling is important in all nasal reconstruction.
- Medical comorbidities and smoking may compromise skin flap.
- Wound size, depth, and location will dictate reconstructive options.
  - Alar reconstruction may require non-anatomic cartilage grafting to replace the uniquely resilient fibrofatty tissue and maintain external nasal valve support.

- Full thickness nasal defects generally require additional flaps or grafts for nasal lining.
- It is reported that this flap can be utilized even in the setting of facial artery ligation (e.g., during neck dissection), but in these cases, one may consider harvest from the contralateral side or utilization of retrograde flow by basing the flap superiorly [7].
- History of radiation should also be considered. In the setting of prior radiation, a thicker axial pattern flap or a different reconstructive option may be considered.

Special Instruments and Positioning

- Handheld Doppler is helpful to trace the vascular pedicle.
- Double prong skin hooks are useful in tissue retraction.

Modifications

- Depending on extent of resection and reconstruction, the flap may be performed as an office-based procedure under local anesthesia.
- Can be performed as a one-stage transposition flap or a two-stage interpolated flap. Interpolated flaps include:
  - Interpolated subcutaneous tissue pedicle.
    - Subcutaneous fat pedicle may have improved vascular and lymphatic function.
    - Pedicle division results in less distortion of the new melolabial crease [4].
  - Interpolated cutaneous pedicle.
    - Allows for thin pedicle (width of 1.5–2.0 cm) [8].
  - Superiorly based interpolated flap.
    - Hinge design can be used for nasal lining.
- Can be unilaterally or bilaterally harvested.
- Variations in the flap design include inferiorly, superiorly, or centrally based pedicles.
- Flap can be supercharged by raising the flap followed by delayed use in reconstruction to improve vascularity.
- Columella reconstruction is possible with cartilage struts folded into the distal portion of the flap. This technique may require bilateral melolabial flaps.
- Flap can be raised and tunneled superiorly into the oral cavity for oronasal fistula repair [9].
- Flap can be raised and tunneled inferiorly for floor of mouth reconstruction.
- Melolabial flaps can be harvested based on random or axial pattern blood supply.
  - Inferiorly based melolabial axial flaps are primarily based off the facial artery. Superiorly based melolabial axial flaps are based on reverse flow from the angular artery [10, 11].
  - In contrast to random pattern harvest, axial pattern melolabial flaps are raised deep to the subcutaneous tissue and include muscle.

Pitfalls and Complications

- Distal flap necrosis can occur due to random blood supply relying on the subdermal vascular plexus.
- Concern for distortion of the alar facial sulcus, which can be potentially avoided by designing an interpolated flap [12]. However, interpolated flaps require a second-stage procedure.
- Subcutaneous fat pedicle requires wide dissection with at least 3 mm depth of fat [4].
- Excess flap thickness may require additional procedure for flap thinning.
- Scarring is a greater concern among younger patients with minimal melolabial crease.
- Medial ectropion can occur if incision is not optimized. Start flap design at least 5 mm below the medial canthus to avoid ectropion [13].
- Upper lip weakness and numbness may result from ligation of nerves and division of muscles but is often minor with unilateral flap harvest.

- Concern for nasal aesthetic and function including subjective nasal obstruction, alar rim retraction, and alar collapse [14].

Postoperative Care

- Keep wound clean and free of crust with ointment.
- Absorbable sutures can be used to avoid suture removal, otherwise non-resorbable sutures can be removed on postoperative day 7.
- Second-stage procedure can be performed 3 weeks after first stage, and up to 4–6 weeks in smokers.
- Wait at least 3 months after completion of reconstruction for flap contouring to allow resolution of swelling.
- Scar care.
  - Avoid sun exposure with physical barrier and/or sunblock.
  - Silicone-based scar gel or sheeting can improve scar appearance starting 2 weeks postoperatively.
  - Hypertrophic scarring can be treated with triamcinolone acetonide (10 mg/mL) starting 6 weeks postoperatively [4]. Injections can be repeated every 4–6 weeks.
  - Dermabrasion, laser resurfacing, or intense pulsed light therapy can be considered 1 year postoperatively [4].

Tissue type: *Cutaneous, fasciocutaneous, myocutaneous*
Artery: *Dermal plexus and perforators from the facial (including angular), infraorbital, and transverse facial artery*
Vein: *Dermal plexus from facial and infraorbital vein*
Nerve: *None*
Flap reach: *Lower and middle third of nose, floor of mouth*
Flap size: *Maximum reported 3.5 cm in width × 9 cm in length* [13]

Operative Procedure

1. Melolabial crease is marked while the patient is awake. Template of the defect is made with the medial border of the flap within the melolabial or nasofacial groove.
   * Doppler can be useful for identification of the artery and design of flap.
   * Injection of local anesthetic. Can consider infraorbital block, especially if performing under local anesthesia.
2. Incise through the skin, dermis, subcutaneous tissue down to the facial muscles. Depth of dissection will vary based on whether harvested as a random or axial pattern flap (Fig. 6.1).
   * Random pattern flaps are thin in design for optimal aesthetic result.
   * Axial pattern flaps require deeper dissection and incorporate the muscles of facial expression into the flap. The perforator artery can be identified.
3. The flap is elevated starting distally and elevating toward the vascular pedicle either in the subcutaneous plane (random pattern) or deep to the facial musculature (axial pattern).
4. Harvested tissue is inset into the defect.
   I. Transposition flap:
   - Flap can be designed to be smaller (approximately two-thirds the diameter) than the defect.
   - Flap is rotated and/or advanced to the defect.
   - Donor site is closed primarily, hiding the incision line in the melolabial fold.

   * Most useful for defects of the nasal sidewall.

   II. Interpolated flap:
   - Island of melolabial skin is pedicled on subcutaneous fat and brought to the nasal defect.
   - Medial edge of the skin should lie within the melolabial crease.
   - A triangle of skin is designed superiorly, avoiding any distortion of the nasal facial

sulcus. This skin can be left on the pedicle until the time of pedicle division. An inferior triangle of skin is excised and discarded to allow a straight-line closure.
- If nasal lining and/or cartilage are required, these are inset prior to insetting the melolabial flap.
- Pedicle take-down occurs 3 weeks later. This can be delayed in patients with a history of radiation or smoking.

  * Most useful for defects of the nasal alar area not involving the nasal facial sulcus.

III. Cutaneous hinge flap:
- Flap can be designed to be transposed 180 degrees to the nasal mucosa. Over time, the skin will mucosalize.

  * Most useful to replace the nasal lining.

5. Close the donor site in a layered fashion.

   * Advance the lateral skin in a superior and medial direction to avoid distortion of the lower eyelid.

   * When necessary, additional contouring of the flap can be performed under local anesthesia after 3 months.

Disclosure Statement No conflicts of interest to disclose.

References

1. Pers M. Cheek flaps in partial Rhinoplasty: a new variation: the in-and-out flap. Scand J Plast Reconstr Surg. 1967;1(1):37–44.
2. Goyal K, Swick M, Mattox A, Pelster MW, Maher IA. Cheek interpolation flaps: a review of the uses and execution of melolabial and paranasal interpolation flaps. Dermatol Surg. 2021;47(2):200–5. https://doi.org/10.1097/DSS.0000000000002621.
3. Rahpeyma A, Khajehahmadi S. The place of nasolabial flap in orofacial reconstruction: a review. Ann Med Surg (Lond). 2016;(12):79–87. https://doi.org/10.1016/j.amsu.2016.11.008.
4. Yellin SA, Nugent A. Melolabial flaps for nasal reconstruction. Facial Plast Surg Clin North Am. 2011;19(1):123–39. https://doi.org/10.1016/j.fsc.2010.10.010.
5. Hynes B, Boyd JB. The nasolabial flap. Axial or random? Arch Otolaryngol Head Neck Surg. 1988;114(12):1389–91. https://doi.org/10.1001/archotol.1988.01860240039019.
6. Whetzel TP, Mathes SJ. Arterial anatomy of the face: an analysis of vascular territories and perforating cutaneous vessels. Plast Reconstr Surg. 1992;89(4):591–603; discussion 604–5.
7. Singh S, Singh RK, Pandey M. Nasolabial flap reconstruction in oral cancer. World J Surg Oncol. 2012;10:227. https://doi.org/10.1186/1477-7819-10-227.
8. Jewett BS. Interpolated forehead and melolabial flaps. Facial Plast Surg Clin North Am. 2009;17(3):361–77. https://doi.org/10.1016/j.fsc.2009.04.003.
9. Schneider B, Pfaffeneder-Mantai F, Grun P, Meller O, Dobbertin K, Turhani D. Melolabial interpolated Island flap for reconstruction of an anterior oronasal fistula after horseshoe Le fort I osteotomy with iliac bone grafts interposition – a case report. Int J Surg Case Rep. 2022;93:106939. https://doi.org/10.1016/j.ijscr.2022.106939.
10. Rose EH. One-stage arterialized nasolabial Island flap for floor of mouth reconstruction. Ann Plast Surg. 1981;6(1):71–5. https://doi.org/10.1097/00000637-198101000-00012.
11. Le-Quang C. Reversed vascular full-thickness nasolabial flap. Ann Chir Plast Esthet. 1994;38(3):273–8.
12. Baker SR, Johnson TM, Nelson BR. The importance of maintaining the alar-facial sulcus in nasal reconstruction. Arch Otolaryngol Head Neck Surg. 1995;121(6):617–22. https://doi.org/10.1001/archotol.1995.01890060015003.
13. Roth J, Patete M, Goodwin WJ. Use of the melolabial flap in intraoral reconstruction. Otolaryngol Head Neck Surg. 1996;114(1):12–7. https://doi.org/10.1016/S0194-59989670276-0.
14. Arden RL, Miguel GS. The subcutaneous melolabial Island flap for nasal alar reconstruction: a clinical review with nuances in technique. Laryngoscope. 2012;122(8):1685–9. https://doi.org/10.1002/lary.23377.

Palatal Island Flap

7

R. Grant Muller and David H. Ludlow

History

- First described by Veau in 1922 and later, in the United States, by Millard in 1962 [1, 2].
- Originally described as a palatal-lengthening technique in children with cleft palate, its use remained limited by findings of resultant craniofacial maldevelopment within this population [2]. However, in 1977, Gullane and Arena repurposed the palatal island flap for use in post-ablative reconstruction in adults [3].

Indications and Benefits

- Reconstruction of oral cavity (hard palate, buccal mucosa, posterior floor of mouth, retromolar trigone) and oropharynx (tonsillar fossa, lateral oropharyngeal wall, soft palate) defects [4].
- Reconstruction of defects up to 4 cm in size.
  - Can be used in combination with other locoregional or free flaps for larger defects.
- Sensate tissue returns function to reconstructed area.
- Single-staged technique that does not require microvascular anastomosis.
- Rich and reliable vascular supply.
- Minimal donor site morbidity.
  - Donor site heals by secondary intention as hard palate re-mucosalizes with little to no contracture.

Anatomy

- Mucoperiosteal flap with keratinized mucosa.
- Hard palate mucosa is firmly attached to the periosteum, which in turn adheres to the palatal bone via fibrous tissue pegs called Sharpey fibers.
- Vascular supply to the palatal island flap is via the greater palatine artery (Fig. 7.1).
  - Greater palatine artery is a branch of the maxillary artery via the descending palatine artery and contributes to both the hard palate and nasal septum.
  - While the greater palatine arteries occur on both right and left sides of the body, the

R. G. Muller
Ear, Nose and Throat Institute, University Hospitals Cleveland Medical Center, Cleveland, OH, USA

Case Western Reserve University School of Medicine, Cleveland, OH, USA

West Cancer Center and Research Institute, Germantown, TN, USA

D. H. Ludlow (✉)
Case Western Reserve University School of Medicine, Cleveland, OH, USA

MetroHealth Medical Center, Cleveland, OH, USA
e-mail: dludlow@metrohealth.org

R. Rezaee, A. Tamaki (eds.), *Local, Regional, and Free Flaps for Head and Neck Reconstruction*,
https://doi.org/10.1007/978-3-032-03211-9_7

palatal island flap is typically based unilaterally.
- Pedicle traverses a bony canal, the greater palatine foramen.
  - Greater palatine foramen is located laterally on the hard palate opposite of the second molar.
- Artery is accompanied by veins and sensory nerves.
  - Greater palatine nerve is a branch of the trigeminal nerve (V2) and allows for a sensate flap.

Preoperative Care

- Assess for history or scars from prior incident or intervention that could have compromised the pedicle (e.g., palatal surgery, ligation of the ipsilateral maxillary or external carotid artery, radiation to palate, or intranasal drug use).
- Contraindicated in patients <5 years.
  - In this population, the maxilla is immature and disruption of the periosteum restricts midface growth resulting in malocclusion [2].

Special Instruments and Positioning

- Mouth gag (e.g., Dingman retractor) to provide adequate exposure for raising and insetting flap.
  - Nasal intubation not required as wide exposure is usually obtained with oral intubation and use of the Dingman or similar retractor.

Modifications

- Flap may be harvested as a random pattern flap rather than a pedicled flap [5].
  - This is useful in areas where rotation is hindered by the pedicle (e.g., third molar region).
  - Flap should not cross midline or exceed a 2.4:1 width-to-length ratio.
  - Flaps of this design should be used with caution due to reduced reliability when not based on the defined pedicle.
- A submucosal variant of the flap can also be raised to alleviate some of the pain associated with this flap.
  - After raising a mucoperiosteal island flap, the mucosa is then separated from underlying submucosal connective tissue, which is rotated into the defect.
  - Mucosa is returned to its native position, covering the exposed maxilla.
- Palatal island flaps can be used in combination with other flaps to reconstruct complex oral and nasal defects [6].

Pitfalls and Complications

- Partial or total flap loss.
- Hemorrhage from the contralateral neurovascular bundle or descending palatine foramen [7].
  - If size of flap warrants, the contralateral greater palatine artery must be ligated for adequate mobilization.
  - The descending palatine artery in the incisive foramen may also require ligation.

Postoperative Care

- Several approaches to management of the donor site can be used:
  - Surgeons can leave the palate to heal by secondary intention, which may contribute significantly to pain.
  - The bone can be covered with a bolster, often made of petroleum-impregnated gauze, and sutured in place.
  - Prefabricated stents or mouth guards can be made to cover the hard palate, taking care not to compress the vascular pedicle.
- Liquid diet is recommended on postoperative day 1 and can then be advanced to a soft diet as tolerated.
- Good oral hygiene should be maintained postoperatively with chlorhexidine mouthwash.
- Patients who smoke should refrain during the

postoperative period as this can contribute to pain and prolonged healing time.

- Complete mucosalization of the hard palate will take 3–5 weeks.

Tissue type: *Mucoperiosteal*
Artery: *Greater palatine artery*
Vein: *Greater palatine vein*
Nerve: *Greater palatine nerve (branch of second division of trigeminal nerve)*
Pedicle length: *The flap can be rotated as much as 180° and reliably reach the soft palate, ipsilateral retromolar trigone, buccal mucosa, and even the tonsillar fossa and lateral oropharyngeal wall*
Flap size: *Approximately 75–90% of the hard palate can be harvested for 16 cm² of surface area of flap*

Operative Procedure

1. Oral intubation is typically preferred when palatal island flap reconstructions are planned. Wide exposure of the oral cavity, particularly the palate, can be achieved with use of a Dingman retractor.
2. A template of the defect can help in the design of the flap; however, to facilitate a tension-free closure it is important to design a flap wider and longer than the size of the defect.
3. Identify the greater palatine foramen through manual palpation of the palate just medial to the second maxillary molar. Doppler may also be useful to confirm location and assess blood flow of the pedicle. In most cases the flap will be based off a unilateral neurovascular pedicle. The incisions are planned lateral to the vessels but at least 3–5 mm medial to the teeth (if present) (Fig. 7.1).

   * In edentulous patients, the flap can be elevated to the maxillary alveolar crest [8].
4. As desired by the surgeon, a vasoconstrictive agent may be injected. A full thickness incision is then carried to the bone with the use of a scalpel or a protected needle tip monopolar cautery device.
5. Raise the flap from anterior to posterior, using a periosteal elevator to release the underlying

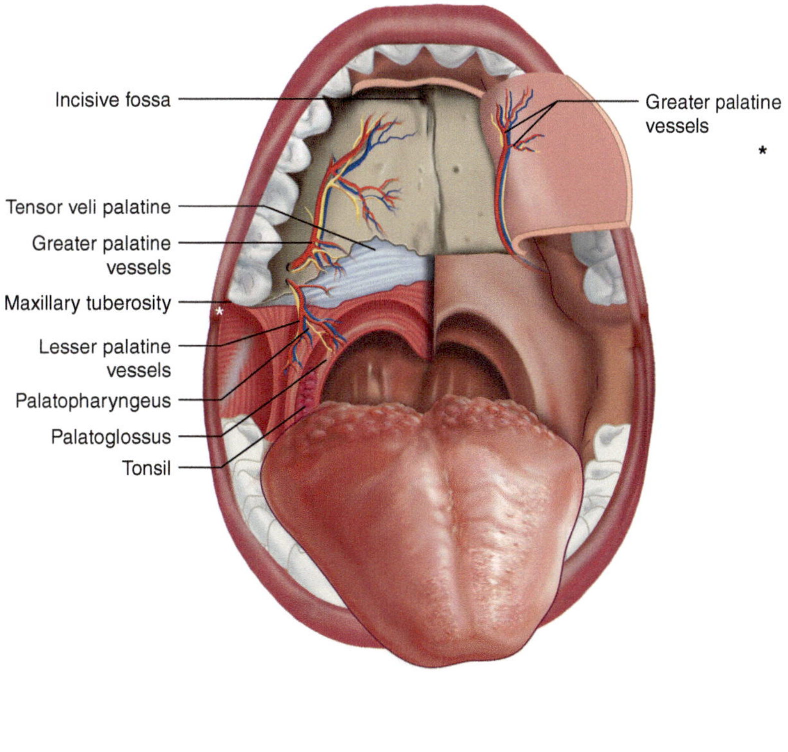

Fig. 7.1 Palatal island flap based off the left greater palatine artery is depicted. The mucoperiosteal flap is elevated from the palatal bone. The structures of the soft palate are shown. The contralateral greater palatine vessels are shown intact in this figure to show anatomy, but would be ligated during full palatal harvest

Sharpey fibers until the vascular pedicle is identified.

* Elevating from the contralateral side first with ligation of the contralateral neurovascular pedicle helps improve visualization and protects vessels.

* It is recommended to ligate the contralateral pedicle and descending palatine artery with suture to prevent retraction of the proximal end of the vessels [7].

6. Additional dissection beyond the foramen is done carefully, frequently checking the flap's mobility. So that the flap may more freely rotate into the defect, prudent back cuts may be necessary.

   * Up to 1 cm increase in the reach and arc of rotation of the flap can be obtained by fracturing the hook of the hamulus or drilling out the posterior wall of the greater palatine foramen.

7. The flap is inset into the defect. Caution is taken to ensure adequate release of the flap to avoid compromise of the vascular pedicle.

   * It is possible to tunnel this flap under mucosa into nonadjacent defects if care is taken not to compress the pedicle.

   * Flap can be rotated across intervening mucosa, although this necessitates a second-stage division of the pedicle 3 or more weeks later.

8. Cover the donor site with exposed palatal bone with a soft stent or xeroform gauze sutured to the palate. The donor site can also be allowed to heal by secondary intention.

Disclosure Statement No conflicts of interest to disclose.

References

1. Veau V, Borel S. Division palatine: anatomie, chirurgie, phonetique; avec la collaboration de S. Borel: Masson; 1931.
2. Millard D. Wide and or short cleft palate. Plast Reconstruct Surg Transplant Bull. 1962;29:40.
3. Gullane PJ, Arena S. Palatal Island flap for reconstruction of oral defects. Arch Otolaryngol. 1977;103:598–9.
4. Gullane PJ, Arena S. Extended palatal Island mucoperiosteal flap. Arch Otolaryngol. 1985;111(5):330–2.
5. Lee JJ, Kok SH, Chang HH, et al. Repair of oroantral communications in the third molar region by random palatal flap. Int J Oral Maxillofac Surg. 2002;31:677–80.
6. Genden EM, Lee BB, Urken ML. The palatal Island flap for reconstruction of palatal and retromolar trigone defects revisited. Arch Otolaryngol Head Neck Surg. 2001;127(7):837–41.
7. Palatal O'LM, Flap I. Oper Tech Otolaryngol Head Neck Surg. 2019;30(2):151–5.
8. Ward BB. The palatal flap. Oral Maxillofac Surg Clin North Am. 2003;15(4):467–73.

Paramedian Forehead Flap

8

Lindsay M. Olinde and Cyrus C. Rabbani

History

- First accounts of the procedure date back to 700 BC in India as a means of nasal tip repair for nasal tip amputation, which was a commonly practiced punishment for various crimes [1].

Indications and Benefits

- Reconstruction of nasal, orbital, and midface defects.
- Thin and easily contoured tissue with excellent color and texture match for nasal and facial skin.
- Reliable blood supply and flap vascularity.
  - Distal flap failure rare due to abundant, superficial axial blood supply [3].
  - Thinning is accomplished without compromising flap blood supply due to supratrochlear artery location in the subcutaneous/subdermal plane within the distal flap [2].

Anatomy

- The paramedian forehead flap is an interpolated, axial flap based on the supratrochlear artery (Fig. 8.1).
  - Significant collateral blood flow to forehead skin from the supraorbital, superficial temporal, and terminal branches of the angular artery allows for the continued viability of forehead skin after flap harvest.
- The supratrochlear artery courses in the vertical axis 1.7–2.2 cm from the midline, travels for 2 cm vertically and then begins to branch significantly.
  - Terminal branches of the supratrochlear artery become increasingly more superfi-

L. M. Olinde (✉)
Department of Otolaryngology- Head and Neck Surgery, LSU Health Shreveport, Shreveport, LA, USA

C. C. Rabbani
Ear, Nose and Throat Institute, University Hospitals Cleveland Medical Center, Cleveland, OH, USA

Case Western Reserve University School of Medicine, Cleveland, OH, USA
e-mail: Cyrus.Rabbani@UHhospitals.org

R. Rezaee, A. Tamaki (eds.), *Local, Regional, and Free Flaps for Head and Neck Reconstruction*,
https://doi.org/10.1007/978-3-032-03211-9_8

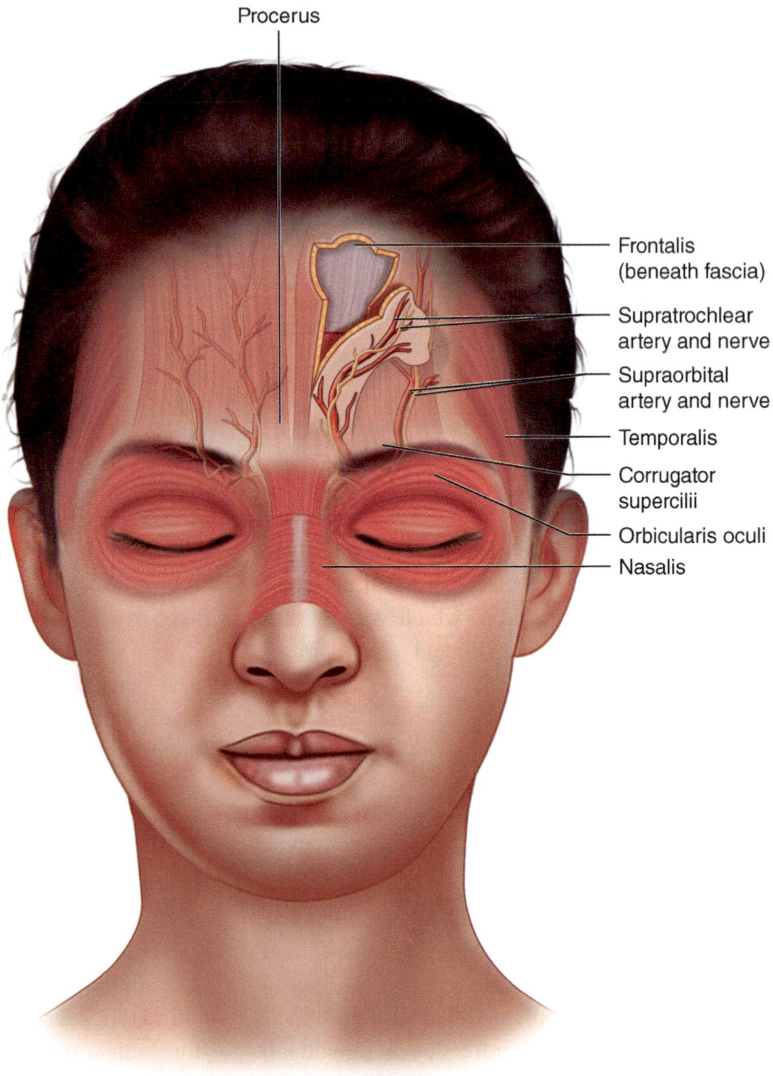

Fig. 8.1 The supratrochlear artery is located 1.7–2.2 cm from the midline. The flap is designed to be approximately 1.5 cm wide at this point to capture the blood supply. When elevating the flap, the dissection should occur in a subgaleal or subfascial plane from superior to inferior. A small portion of the distal flap can be elevated in a subcutaneous plane before transitioning to a subfascial plane. Proximally, elevation should move into a subperiosteal plane, ensuring the vascular pedicle is safely captured 1–2 cm above the supraorbital rim. The hairline often limits the length of the graft

cial until they reach the subdermal plane at the hairline.

- Venous drainage is via the frontal vein.

Preoperative Care

- Careful assessment and measurement of the defect.
  - Nasal defects >1.5–2 cm in the horizontal axis are best suited to repair with a paramedian forehead flap (versus skin grafts or other local advancement flaps) [4].
- Assess the forehead donor site.
  - Note the anterior hairline height and forehead laxity.
  - Note any prior scars and history of prior forehead or orbital trauma and any prior procedures that would disrupt the blood supply.
- Counsel patients regarding appearance during the staged portion of reconstruction and prior to pedicle separation.

Special Instruments and Positioning

- Supine, reverse Trendelenburg position.
- Eye protection (moist eye pads).
- Sterile prep of the full face and superiorly to the mid-vertex scalp.
- Optional use of Doppler probe to localize supratrochlear artery but not required due to anatomic consistency.

Modifications

- Additional length can be added to the vertical height of the flap by obliquely angling the flap toward the temporal recession just inferior to the hairline. This is appropriate for smaller flaps (<3 cm). Too much recruitment of the lateral scalp can lead to excessive scaring or tethering of the lateral brow [5].
- In cases of short foreheads or low hairlines, tissue expansion may be a consideration to avoid hair transfer to the recipient site. This may ultimately create thickening of the epidermis in the skin flap, a trade-off to avoid hair bearing skin.
- It can be used as a lining whenever septal mucoperichondrium or turbinate mucosa is unavailable (e.g., total or near total nasal defects) [6].
- Can be used for total nasal reconstruction.
  - In conjunction with radial forearm free flap or other structural grafts (e.g., cartilage or calvarial bone).
  - It can be harvested in tandem with the contralateral paramedian forehead flap—one flap designed for the internal lining of the nose and one to cover the external defect [1].

Pitfalls and Complications

- Most cases require a second operation for pedicle detachment.
  - Minimum time for neovascularization is 10–14 days. Commonly, pedicle is maintained for 3 weeks (longer for active smokers).
  - Interferes with wearing glasses during this time.
- Development of hematomas under the distal flap due to the prominent vascularity and potential for blood accumulation between distal flap and underlying nasal framework.
- Donor site scar.
  - Difficult to close flaps designed >4.5 cm wide. These are left open to close by secondary intention or skin grafted. Secondary intention provides favorable cosmetic results.
- Hair transfer to the nose from vertex scalp.
  - Can thin skin and cauterize individual hair follicles during the initial operation.

Post Operative Care

- The patient cannot wear glasses during the initial postoperative period.
- Postoperative care to suture line.
- Prevention of desiccation of the pedicle (application of petrolatum-impregnated gauze to the pedicle).
- Schedule pedicle detachment (approximately 3 weeks following initial surgery).

Tissue type: *Fascial, fasciocutaneous*
Artery: *Supratrochlear artery (axial), subdermal plexus (random component)*
Vein: *Frontal vein (supratrochlear vein)*
Nerve: *None*
Pedicle reach: *Upper two-thirds of the face. Maximum pedicle reach limited by supraorbital rim and anterior hairline. Reported to reach the palate*
Flap size: *Can take vast majority of central forehead skin (bilateral paramedian forehead flap). Limitations on size are based on hair-bearing skin. If less than < 4 cm wide, can allow for primary closure of donor site*

Operative Procedure

1. Pedicle is centered over the supratrochlear artery ipsilateral to the nasal defect. The base is designed approximately 1.5 cm wide to

appropriately capture artery and this allows for best arc of rotation (Fig. 8.1).

* Recall the location and course of the artery: oriented in the vertical axis 1.7–2.2 cm from the midline, travels for 2 cm vertically, then begins to branch significantly.

2. A template is designed that replicates the defect to be reconstructed.

   * If cartilage grafts are needed for a full-thickness nasal defect, the template is designed after the placement of the cartilage grafts.

3. The template is placed on the forehead, centered over the axis of the supratrochlear artery (described above). This outline is traced with a skin marker.

   * Avoid placement of the template beyond the hairline, if possible.

   * The template distance from the base of the flap should be measured by mimicking the flap rotation into the recipient site with a gauze sponge or non-stretchable suture material.

   * Adjustments to length can be made by placing the template higher on the forehead or lowering the proximal extent of the pedicle below the level of the eyebrow.

4. Local anesthetic is injected.
5. Incision made through skin, subcutaneous tissue, muscle, and fascia.
6. Flap elevation occurs from superior to inferior in a subgaleal or subfascial plane. A limited portion of the distal aspect of the flap may be elevated in a subcutaneous plane before entering the subfascial plane. Elevation is transitioned to a subperiosteal plane proximally to safely capture the vascular pedicle approximately 1–2 cm above the supraorbital rim. Elevation is completed when satisfactory length is achieved for a tension-free wound closure at the recipient site.

   * At the level of the corrugator supercilii muscle, the muscle is dissected away from the underlying periosteum. Commonly, division of the muscle is necessary to allow adequate flap mobilization.

   * The supratrochlear artery can be visualized on the deep surface of the frontalis muscle as it exits over or through the corrugator supercilii muscle before passing deep to the orbicularis oculi muscle to enter the orbit [1].

7. The distal flap is then thinned to match the thickness of the recipient site.

   * All but the subcutaneous fat immediately attached to the dermis may be removed.

   * Usually more proximal portions of the flap are left with the underlying muscle and subcutaneous tissue intact until the second stage where it can be safely thinned at the time of pedicle division.

   * Any hair follicles transferred with the flap should be individually cauterized or manually removed.

8. The flap is then pivoted in an arc toward the midline and reflected downward to be inset into the defect. Distally, the flap is secured with interrupted cutaneous sutures.

   * The cephalic aspect of the nasal defect will be approximated to the proximal flap at the time of pedicle detachment.

   * Judicious hemostasis of the proximal portion of the flap is performed with electrocautery.

9. A layered closure of the forehead donor site is then performed by extensive undermining in a subfascial plane (can be extended from one temporalis to the other).

   * To facilitate primary closure, parallel vertical galeotomies may be made.

   * Standing cutaneous deformity of the scalp from the advancement of the forehead skin is removed.

   * Drain placement is not necessary.

   * Superior aspect may not close completely (defects >4 cm). This is often left to heal by secondary intension.

10. Subsequent stages of flap contouring and cartilage grafting may be performed to achieve appropriate contour at the recipient site before the division of the pedicle. More aggressive distal flap contouring and thinning can take place prior to division of the pedicle.

Pedicle Division

1. Performed a minimum of 3 weeks following initial procedure. Consider delay in cases of delayed healing (e.g., in the setting of diabetes, smoking, radiation).
2. Local anesthetic injection at pedicle base and cephalic most flap attachment to the nose.
3. Clamp across the pedicle with a hemostat at the superior margin of the defect and separate.
4. Further thinning of the more proximal flap can be performed at this time.
5. Inset of the now released portion with cutaneous, interrupted sutures.
6. The base of the pedicle is returned to its donor site and closed to return the normal intereyebrow distance.

Disclosure Statement No conflicts of interest to disclose.

References

1. Baker SR. Interpolated paramedian forehead flaps. Local flaps in head and neck reconstruction. Philadelphia: Mosby; 2007.
2. Urken ML. Paramedian forehead Atlas of regional and free flaps for head and neck reconstruction. Baltimore/Philadelphia: Lippincott Williams & Wilkins; 2012.
3. Shumrick KA, Smith TL. The anatomic basis for the design of forehead flaps in nasal reconstruction. Arch Otolaryngol Head Neck Surg. 1992;118:373.
4. Larrabee WF, Sherris DA, Teixeira JC. Principles of facial reconstruction: a subunit approach to cutaneous repair. New York: Thieme.
5. Baker SR. Oblique forehead flap for total reconstruction of the nasal tip and columella. Archiv Otolaryngol Head and Neck Surg. 1985;111:425.
6. Tollefson TT, Kriet JD. Complex nasal defects: structure and internal lining. Facial Plastic Surg Clin North Am. 2005;13:2.

9 Partial Lip Reconstruction: Abbe and Estlander Flaps

Eric L. Cole, Jamil Asaria, and Rohan R. Joshi

Introduction

- The lips occupy a central role in facial aesthetics and serve a key functional role in emotional expression as well as oral competence.
- Small defects of the lip (less than one-third of the horizontal width) can be reconstructed via primary closure. Defects larger than one-third of the horizontal width of the lip must employ flap reconstruction techniques.
- This chapter will focus on reconstruction of the lips when defects range from one-third to two-thirds the horizontal width of the lips using two common local flaps: the Abbe flap and Estlander flap.

E. L. Cole
Department of Plastic Surgery, University of Texas Medical Branch, Galveston, TX, USA

J. Asaria
Department of Otolaryngology- Head and Neck Surgery, University of Toronto, FACE Toronto, Toronto, ON, Canada

R. R. Joshi (✉)
Origins Plastic Surgery, Anti-Aging and Wellness, Houston, TX, USA
e-mail: rohan.joshi@originsplasticsurgery.com

Anatomy

- Abbe and Estlander flaps are pedicled on the superior or inferior labial artery of the opposing lip.
- Superior and inferior labial arteries branch from the facial artery.
  - Superior labial artery [1, 2]
    Vertical location is within 1 cm of the free margin of the lip.
      - In the midline, courses inferior to level of the vermillion–cutaneous junction between the orbicularis muscle and wet mucosa 75% of the time; at the commissure, courses at the level vermillion between the orbicularis muscle and wet mucosa 6% of the time.

    Courses between orbicularis oris muscle and wet mucosa the majority of the time but may also course within the orbicularis muscle.
  - Inferior labial artery [1, 2]
    Vertical location is within 1.5 cm of the free margin on the lip.
      - In the midline, courses at the level of the vermillion between the orbicularis muscle and wet mucosa 100% of the time; at the commissure, courses superior to the vermillion–cutaneous junction 80% of the time.

R. Rezaee, A. Tamaki (eds.), *Local, Regional, and Free Flaps for Head and Neck Reconstruction*,
https://doi.org/10.1007/978-3-032-03211-9_9

– Courses between orbicularis oris muscle and wet mucosa the majority of the time, but may also course within the orbicularis muscle.
- Venous drainage is provided by small veins which lie parallel to the labial artery.
  – Flap pedicle should be sufficient enough to allow venous drainage, but thin enough to allow adequate rotation and inset [1].
- Flap width is dependent on two considerations:
  – To maintain proportions between the two lips, the flap may be designed to be one half the width of the defect.
  – When the defect spans an entire subunit such as the philtrum or lateral subunit, consider transferring a flap that is similar in width to the defect [1].

Preoperative Care

- Preoperative history and exam to ensure no previous lip surgery or external carotid system surgery that could compromise the labial artery.

Special Instruments and Positioning

- Contralateral nasal intubation to prevent distortion of the lip and facilitate access.

Pitfalls and Complications

- Contour deformities.
- Inadequate approximation resulting in misaligned vermillion.
- Trap door deformity from restriction of lymphatic drainage due to scar formation.
- Microstomia from decreased oral aperture.
- Risk of denervation.
  – Partial sensory return begins after several months. Reports of regained pain sensation after 2 months, tactile sensation at 3 months, cold sensation at 6 months, and warm sensation at 9 months [3]. Movement does return, but to a variable degree in patients [3, 4]. May result in oral competence issues.
- Estlander flaps can result in blunting of the oral commissure that may require later commissuroplasty.

Postoperative Care

- Patient is allowed to consume liquids and very soft solids that require minimal mastication.
- Abbe flap is sewn into recipient site and left in place for 3 weeks while revascularization occurs.
- Once pedicle is divided, vermillion of donor site and recipient site are aligned, and a four-layer closure is performed.
- Frequently, Estlander flaps may require a later commissuroplasty to address blunting of the neo-commissure.

I. Abbe Flap

History

- Cross-lip transfer, specifically a two-stage cross-lip transfer, was first described by Sabatini in 1838, but later described by Abbe in 1898 [1, 5–7].

Indications and Benefits

- Reconstruction of full thickness lip defects ranging in size from one -third to two-thirds of the width of the upper or lower lip [1, 8].
- Defects medial to the oral commissure.

Modifications

- V, W, or rectangular designs can be created depending on the reconstructive needs [5].
- Bilateral cross lip flap can be taken to distribute tissue loss among upper lip rather than preferentially reduce one side over the other.

When doing so, adhere to the subunit principle and avoid harvesting from the philtrum [9].
- Depending on the degree of tissue loss, can be combined with unilateral or bilateral horizontal advancement flaps.

Tissue type: *Myocutaneous*
Artery: *Labial artery*
Vein: *Venae comitantes*
Nerve: *Motor innervation from facial nerve, sensory innervation from V2 or V3*
Flap reach: *Anatomic extent of the upper or lower lip*
Flap size: *Up to two-thirds the horizontal width of the lip*

Operative Procedure

1. Planned flap is marked out on skin and intraorally (Fig. 9.1). Flap design:
   - To maintain proportions between the two lips, the flap may be designed to be one half the width of the defect.
   - When the defect spans an entire subunit such as the philtrum or lateral subunit, consider transferring a flap that is similar in width to the defect [1].
   - The length of the flap can be smaller than the length of the defect. Primary closure of the distal margin of the defect facilitates this.

   * Flap pedicle should be sufficiently thick enough to allow venous drainage, but thin enough to allow adequate rotation and inset [1].

   * Local anesthetic using 1% lidocaine with 1:100,000 epinephrine is used circumferentially around planned incision sites. Care is taken around the pedicle.

   * Methylene blue or gentian violet can be used to mark the vermillion–cutaneous lip border using a 25- or 27-gauge needle.
2. Incision is made through the skin on the non-pedicled side. This is carried down to and through the orbicularis muscle. The labial artery should be identified and ligated in some manner (suture or cautery). The lip is then turned over and the incision is completed through the mucosa.
3. Incision is made on the pedicled side up to the vermillion. The incision is carried through skin, orbicularis muscle, and mucosa up to the vicinity of the vermillion. The location of the labial artery on the non-pedicled side should provide some insight as to its location on the pedicled side. A cuff of tissue around the labial artery is needed for venous drainage. Care should be taken with the intraoral incision as the labial artery may be just deep to the mucosa. A pedicle of approximately 1.5 cm is left on the intraoral surface of the lip.

   * In some instances, incision through the vermillion for 3–4 mm is necessary to allow for increased rotation. However, at least 5 mm must be left intact to allow adequate blood flow to the vermillion [8].

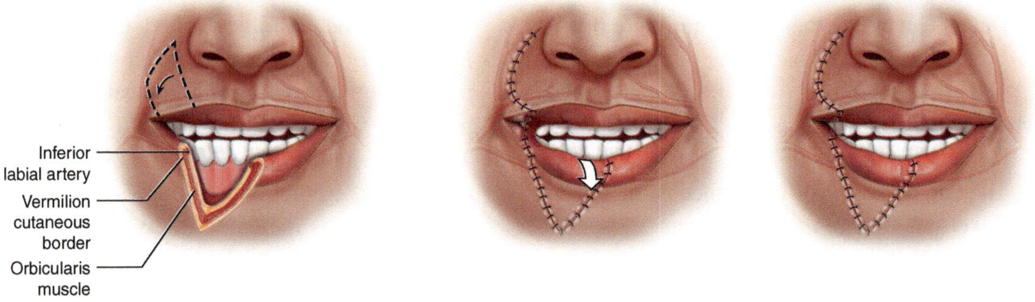

Fig. 9.1 Abbe flap procedural steps. The three photos demonstrate flap and flap rotation into a commissure-sparing defect. Note the medially based pedicle

4. Flap is rotated 180 degrees and sutured in place at the recipient site.
5. The orbicularis muscle is reconstituted first. Next, the vermillion–mucosal junction and vermillion–cutaneous junction should be aligned. A full four-layer closure should be performed, approximating orbicularis, intraoral mucosa, deep dermal tissue, and lastly skin. Approximation of the orbicularis muscle is necessary to reconstruct the oral sphincter.
6. The donor site is closed primarily with a full four-layer closure.
7. After 3 weeks (may consider 2 weeks for low-risk patients, 4 weeks for high-risk patients and smokers), the pedicle is lysed and the remaining tissue is inset into the upper and lower lip, taking great care to realign the vermillion. Closure should take place in a four-layer fashion.

II. Estlander Flap

History

- Single-stage cross-lip transfer with the pedicle incorporated into the reconstruction was described by Estlander in 1872 [10].

Indications and Benefits

- Reconstruction of full thickness lip defects ranging in size from one-third to two-thirds of the width of the upper or lower lip [1, 8].
- One-stage reconstruction.
- Defects involving the oral commissure only.

Modifications

- The flap was originally designed as a triangle.
- Baker modification creates a rounded apex to the flap that lies within the melolabial crease.

Tissue type: Myocutaneous
Artery: *Labial artery*
Vein: Venae comitantes
Nerve: Motor innervation from facial nerve, Sensory innervation from V2 or V3
Flap reach: Anatomic extent of the upper or lower lip
Flap size: Up to two-thirds the horizontal width of the lip

Operative Procedure

1. Planned flap is marked out on skin and intraorally (Fig. 9.2). Flap design:
   - Width of planned flap at the vermillion should be one half the width of the defect at the vermillion [11].
   - The length of the flap can be smaller than the length of the defect. Primary closure of the distal margin of the defect facilitates this.

   * Local anesthetic using 1% lidocaine with 1:100,000 epinephrine is used circumferentially around planned incision sites. Care is taken around the pedicle.

   * Methylene blue or gentian violet can be used to mark the vermillion–cutaneous lip border using a 25- or 27-gauge needle.
2. Incision is made through the skin on the non-pedicled side (in this case, the lateral incision). This is carried down to and through the orbicularis muscle. The labial artery should be identified and ligated in some manner (suture or cautery). The lip is then transposed over and the incision is completed through the mucosa.
3. Incision is made on the pedicled side up to the vermillion. The incision is carried through skin, orbicularis muscle, and mucosa up to the vicinity of the vermillion. The location of the labial artery on the non-pedicled side should provide some insight as to its location on the pedicled side. A sufficient cuff of tissue around the labial artery is needed for venous drainage. Care should be taken with the intraoral incision as the labial artery may be just deep to the mucosa. A pedicle of approximately 1.5 cm is left on the intraoral surface of the lip. In some instances, incision through the vermillion for 3–4 mm is necessary to allow for increased rotation. However, at least

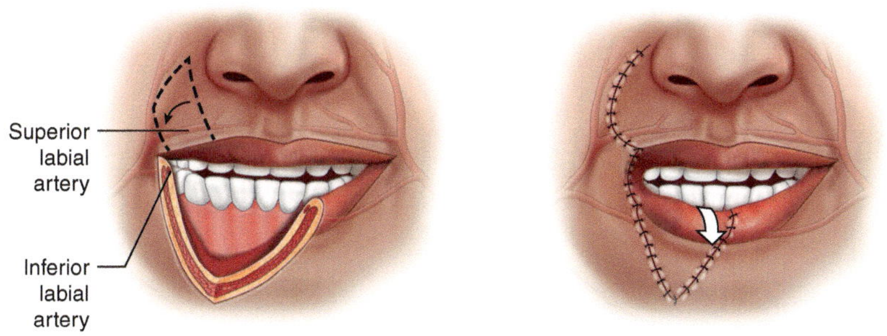

Fig. 9.2 Estlander flap procedural steps. The two photos demonstrate flap and flap rotation into commissure-involving defect. Note the medially based pedicle

5 mm must be left intact to allow adequate blood flow to the vermillion [8].

4. Flap is rotated 180° and sutured in place at the recipient site.
5. The orbicularis muscle is reconstituted first. Next, the vermillion-mucosal junction and vermillion–cutaneous junction should be aligned. A full four-layer closure should be performed, approximating orbicularis, intraoral mucosa, deep dermal tissue, and lastly skin. Approximation of the orbicularis muscle is necessary to reconstruct the oral sphincter.
6. The donor site is closed primarily with a full four-layer closure.

Disclosure Statement No conflicts of interest to disclose.

References

1. Renner G. Reconstruction of the lips. In: Local flaps in facial reconstruction. 3rd ed. Elsevier; 2021. p. 481–529.
2. Schulte DL, Sherris DA, Kasperbauer JL. The Anatomical basis of the Abbé flap: the anatomical basis of the Abbé flap. Laryngoscope. 2001;111(3):382–6. https://doi.org/10.1097/00005537-200103000-00004.
3. Smith JW. The anatomical and physiologic acclimatization of tissue transplanted by the lip switch technique. Plast Reconstr Surg Transplant Bull. 1960;26:40–56. https://doi.org/10.1097/00006534-196007000-00003.
4. Thompson N, Pollard AC. Motor function in Abbe flaps. Br J Plast Surg. 1961;14:66–75. https://doi.org/10.1016/S0007-1226(61)80012-X.
5. Sabatini P. Cenno storico dell'origine e progressi della rinoplastica e cheiloplastica. Bologna Bella Arti. Published online 1838.
6. Abbe R. A new plastic operation for the relief of the deformity due to double harelip. Med Rec. 1889;53
7. Mazzola RF, Lupo G. Evolving concepts in lip reconstruction. Clin Plast Surg. 1984;11(4):583–617.
8. Shokri T, Lighthall JG. Lip reconstruction using the Sabattini-Abbé cross-lip flap. Oper Tech Otolaryngol Head Neck Surg. 2020;31(1):13–7. https://doi.org/10.1016/j.otot.2019.12.004.
9. Williams EF, Chaiet SR. Lip reconstruction. In: Facial plastic and reconstructive surgery. 4th ed. Thieme; 2016. p. 718–29.
10. Estlander J. Eine Methode aus der einen Lippe Substanzverluste der anderen zu ersetzen. Arch Klin Chir. 1872;14
11. Eggerstedt M, Smith RM, Revenaugh PC. Estlander flap for lip reconstruction. Oper Tech Otolaryngol Head Neck Surg. 2020;31(1):10–2. https://doi.org/10.1016/j.otot.2019.12.003.

Pectoralis Major Flap

10

Chelsea S. Hamill and Pierre Lavertu

History

- The pectorals muscle flap was first introduced as a turnover flap for chest reconstruction by Pickrell in 1947 [1].
- It gained widespread acceptance with Arnold and Pairolero's major contributions to chest wall reconstruction in the 1970s and 1980s [1].
- First introduced for head and neck reconstruction by Ariyan et al. in 1979 [2].

Indications and Benefits

- Useful for reconstruction of:
  - Mucosal defects (oral cavity, oropharynx, larynx, pharynx).
  - Cutaneous defects (neck, parotid).
  - Salvage laryngectomy defects.
  - Vascular coverage to prevent carotid ruptures after chemoradiation.
  - Fistula coverage after free flap failure.
  - Patients with a vessel depleted neck.
- Regional tissue option located outside of the radiation field [3, 4].
- Short operating time.
- Versatile with myocutaneous and myofascial flap options.
- Robust blood supply and consistent vascular anatomy leading to increased reliability.

Anatomy

- The pectoralis muscle has five points of origin: the anterior surface of the medial half of the clavicle, anterior surface of the sternum, first seven costal cartilages, sternal end of the sixth rib, and aponeurosis of the external oblique [5].
- The pectoralis muscle fibers converge onto one insertion point: the intertubercular sulcus of the humerus [5].
- There are two heads to the pectoralis muscle: the sternal and clavicular heads [5].
  - The clavicular head is innervated by the lateral pectoral nerve.
  - The sternal head is innervated by the medial pectoral nerve.
- The pectoral artery arises from the thoracoacromial trunk, the second branch of the axillary

C. S. Hamill
Department of Otolaryngology- Head and Neck Surgery, University of Nebraska Medical Center, Omaha, NE, USA

P. Lavertu (✉)
Ear, Nose and Throat Institute, University Hospitals Cleveland Medical Center, Cleveland, OH, USA

Case Western Reserve University School of Medicine, Cleveland, OH, USA
e-mail: pierre.lavertu@uhhospitals.org

R. Rezaee, A. Tamaki (eds.), *Local, Regional, and Free Flaps for Head and Neck Reconstruction*, https://doi.org/10.1007/978-3-032-03211-9_10

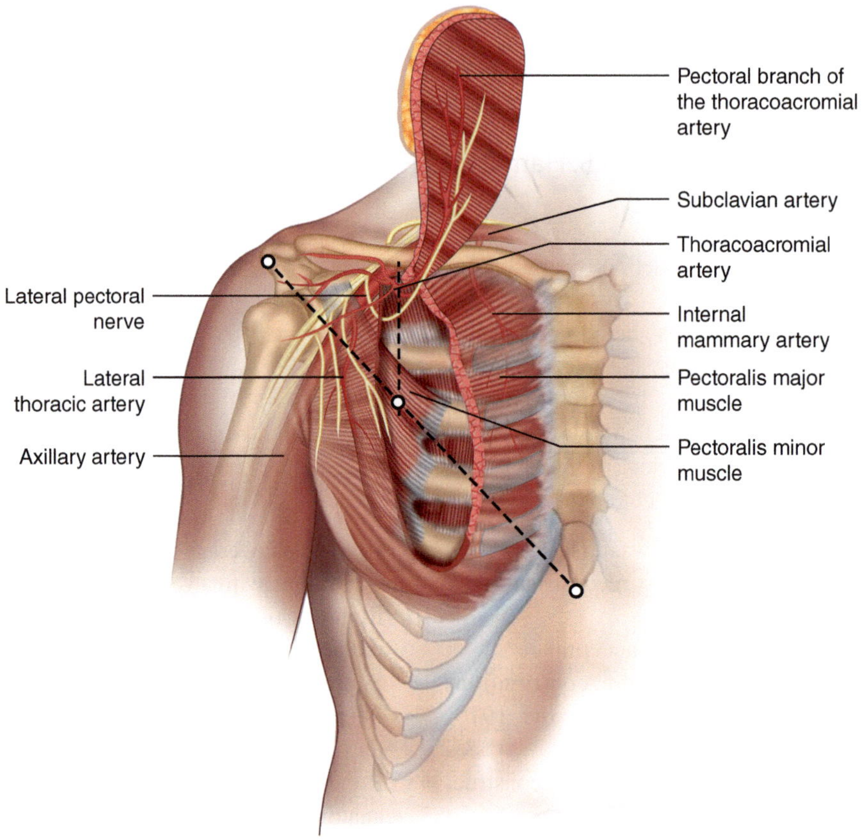

Fig. 10.1 The pectoralis major regional flap is seen raised with a skin paddle and portion of the pectoralis major muscle. Arterial supply is from the pectoral branch of the thoracoacromial artery. The course of the vascular pedicle is along an axis drawn from the acromion to the xiphoid process. The crossing point between a second perpendicular line from the distal third of the clavicle is used as the superior limit of the skin paddle

artery [5]. This runs within a fascial plane on the deep surface of the pectoralis muscle (Fig. 10.1).

- The pectoral vein drains into the subclavian vein.
- The anterior cutaneous branches of the intercostal nerves supply the skin over the anterior chest [4].
- The pectoralis minor muscle lies deep to the pectoralis major [6].

Preoperative Care

- Assess for history of or scars from prior surgery or trauma that may compromise vascular anatomy or perfusion to the skin (e.g., pacemaker, breast implant, implanted port).
- Shave any hair-bearing skin in male patients prior to prepping for surgery if planning on myocutaneous option.

Special Instruments and Positioning

- Patients can remain in the supine position with exposure of the chest from the contralateral sternal border, inferior to the xyphoid, and laterally to the shoulder and mid-axillary line.
- Position with or without a shoulder roll in place.

Modifications

- Can extend the skin paddle up to 2.5 cm inferior to the pectoralis muscle and raise with underlying fascia, creating a random flap blood supply.
- Consider inframammary incision in female patients for myofascial flaps.
- Can be harvested as myofascial only flap.
  - If the muscle is exposed and requires coverage, a full or split thickness skin graft (0.12–0.20 inch thickness) can be used.
- Can be harvested with segment of costal cartilage or lateral portion of the anterior cortex of the sternum [4].
- Has potential to be harvested as a free flap with pedicle length of 9 cm with an artery of 4 mm and vein of 5 mm diameter [7].

Pitfalls and Complications

- If a cutaneous portion is needed in an obese patient, may have excess bulky soft tissue overlying the muscle [8].
- May distort the breast in female patients.
- Contraindications:
  - Prior chest surgery
  - Defects superior to the zygomatic arch
  - Congenital absence of pectoralis muscle, such as in Poland syndrome [4]
- Ensure all muscle perforators are ligated/controlled as the humeral attachment is taken down to prevent hematoma in the axilla.
- Ensure all internal mammary artery perforators are ligated properly with clips or suture to prevent retraction and hemothorax formation.
- Mild to moderate shoulder pain and dysfunction [4].

Postoperative Care

- Two closed suction drains within the cavity. One should lay along the medial aspect and the second into the axilla. Both should exit inferiorly to allow for dependent drainage.
- Monitor drain output and chest incision for seroma or hematoma formation.
- Alert nursing staff as to the baseline appearance if bulky at the level of the clavicle.
- Avoid external pressure or circumferential ties at the level of the low neck as the vascular pedicle can risk potential compression at its crossing point over the clavicle.

Tissue type: *Myocutaneous, myofascial*
Artery: *Pectoral branch of thoracoacromial artery*
Vein: *Pectoral vein*
Nerve: *Medial and lateral pectoral nerves*
Flap reach: *Reported to reach up to the zygomatic arch*
Flap size: *Muscle averages 15 cm (12–22 cm) length × 24 cm (21–26 cm) width* [8]. *Skin averages 12 cm (7–20 cm) length × 8 cm (5–22 cm) width* [8, 9]

Operative Procedure

1. If performing a myocutaneous flap, design a skin paddle to the desired dimensions. Mark a curvilinear incision from the proximal aspect of the skin paddle along the chest extending to the clavicle toward the pedicle location (Fig. 10.1).

   * *Course of the vascular pedicle is along an axis drawn from the acromion to the xiphoid process.*

   * Place medial to the nipple in men. In women can place within the inframammary crease to minimize excess bulk from breast tissue.
2. Ensure the distal aspect of the skin paddle reaches the defect by utilizing a towel or lap "pedicled" on the clavicle ending at the skin paddle and rotated superiorly to the defect.

3. Incise the skin on the lateral aspect of the skin paddle up to the clavicle. Carry down through the subcutaneous tissue down to the fascia overlying the pectoralis muscle. Raise a suprafascial flap laterally until the lateral edge of the pectoralis muscle is identified.

   * Consider securing the skin paddle down to the muscle to prevent sheering of the perforators as the flap is being raised and manipulated.
4. In a similar fashion, incise the skin on the medial aspect of the skin paddle and carry down to the pectoralis muscle fascia. Raise a suprafascial flap medially until the sternum and the medial border of the muscle is visualized.
5. Continue to raise a skin flap superiorly extending over the clavicle and connect a tunnel into the neck. Ensure the width of this tunnel is 4 fingerbreadths.
6. Identify the lateral border of the pectoralis major muscle and separate from the underlying pectoralis minor muscle using blunt dissection.
7. While providing retraction on the muscle, divide the muscular attachments from the ribs and sternum with Bovie electrocautery or advanced energy device.

   * Divide the muscle along the costochondral junction to prevent violation of the internal mammary artery perforators. If encountered, ligate these vessels with clips to prevent retraction and hemothorax formation.
8. Once elevated, identify the pedicle within the deep fascia of the underlying surface of the pectoralis major muscle. Divide any branches from the lateral thoracic artery to the pectoralis minor.
9. While keeping the pedicle in view, divide the humeral attachments of the pectoralis major.
10. Identify the medial pectoral nerves and divide for additional mobility of the flap and denervation of the posterolateral portion of the sternal head. This nerve has a more variable course but, in general, it pierces the pectoralis minor at the level of the third intercostal before entering the pectoralis major. Next, the lateral pectoral nerve should be identified and ligated. The lateral pectoral nerve runs a more constant course along the deep surface of the muscle with the vascular pedicle. This should denervate the superior sternal and clavicular head.

    * Ligating these nerves help to decrease excess bulk over time.
11. To add an additional 1-cm, divide the medial attachment of the muscle to the clavicle. This will also minimize bulk over the clavicle.
12. Pass the flap through the previously dissected tunnel, ensure the pedicle is not twisted. Secure the flap into the defect requiring reconstruction.
13. Ensure hemostasis is obtained in the chest and place two suction drains. Close the chest wall primarily in a layered fashion.

Disclosure Statement No conflicts of interest to disclose.

References

1. Bakri K, Mardini S, Evans KK, Carlsen BT, Arnold PG. Workhorse flaps in chest wall reconstruction: the pectoralis major, latissimus dorsi, and rectus abdominis flaps. Semin Plast Surg. 2011;25(1):43–54.
2. Ariyan S. The pectoralis major myocutaneous flap. Plast Reconstr Surg. 1979;63:73–81.
3. Liu M, Liu W, Yang X, Guo H, Peng H. Pectoralis major Myocutaneous flap for head and neck defects in the era of free flaps: harvesting technique and indications. Sci Rep. 2017;7:46256.
4. Pectoralis Major Flap. In: Plastic surgery key. WordPress; 2019. 7. 2018. https://plasticsurgerykey.com/pectoralis-major-flap/#
5. Solari F, Burns B. Anatomy, Thorax, Pectoralis Major. [Updated 2022 Jul 25]. In: StatPearls [Internet]. Treasure Island (FL): StatPearls Publishing; 2022 Jan-. Available from: https://www.ncbi.nlm.nih.gov/books/NBK525991/
6. Baig MA, Bordoni B. Anatomy, Shoulder and Upper Limb, Pectoral Muscles. [Updated 2022 Aug 30]. In: StatPearls [Internet]. Treasure Island (FL): StatPearls Publishing; 2023. Available from: https://www.ncbi.nlm.nih.gov/books/NBK545241/
7. Trainotti S, Hoffmann TK, Rotter N, et al. Pectoralis major muscle free flap: anatomical studies on pedicle length and vessel diameter. Ear Nose Throat J. 2019;98(7):431–4.
8. Shah JP, Haribhakti V, Loree TR, Sutaria P. Complications of the pectoralis major myocutaneous flap in head and neck reconstruction. Am J Surg. 1990;160(4):352–5.
9. Konduru V, Tirkey AJ, Samy K, Devarakonda KK, Janakiraman R. The folded, bipaddled pectoralis major myocutaneous flap for complex oral cavity defects: undiminished relevance in the era of free flaps. JPRAS Open. 2020;25(27):108–18.

11 Submental Island Flap

Marisa R. Buchakjian and Rodrigo Bayon

History

- First described by Martin et al. in 1993 [1] as a regional flap with superior arc of rotation, donor site morbidity, and recipient site options compared to traditional cervical rotational flaps.

Indications and Benefits

- Reconstruction of oral cavity, cutaneous, pharynx, and lateral skull base defects.
  - Useful in auriculectomy and lateral temporal bone defects.
  - Useful in oral cavity defects such as oral tongue and floor or mouth as an alternative to free flap reconstruction.
- Thin, pliable tissue with excellent color match for cutaneous defects.
  - Thickness may be modified based on reconstructive needs by harvesting mylohyoid and contralateral anterior belly of digastric muscle to increase bulk.
- Axial patterned flap with reliable and familiar vascular pedicle anatomy.
  - The submental artery is a consistent branch of the facial artery. Location of the submental artery relative to the submandibular gland and anterior belly of digastric is variable and requires careful intraoperative dissection.
- Maximal flap width is dependent on patient skin laxity but may be as large as 7 cm. Flap length may extend from mandibular angle to mandibular angle depending on tissue size and arc of rotation needed.

Anatomy

- Axial patterned flap based on perforators from the submental artery.
- Submental artery is a 1.0–1.5 mm caliber vessel, which is a consistent branch of the facial artery. The submental artery branches from the facial artery at the posterolateral aspect of the submandibular gland and travels medially toward the anterior belly of digastric, parallel to the inferior border of the mandible (Fig. 11.1).
- Submental artery may run deep (70%) or superficial (30%) to the anterior belly of digastric and run superficial to the mylohyoid muscle [2].

M. R. Buchakjian
Department of Otolaryngology- Head and Neck Surgery, University of Michigan, Ann Arbor, MI, USA

R. Bayon (✉)
Department of Otolaryngology- Head and Neck Surgery, University of Iowa Hospitals and Clinics, Iowa City, IA, USA
e-mail: Rodrigo-Bayon@uiowa.edu

R. Rezaee, A. Tamaki (eds.), *Local, Regional, and Free Flaps for Head and Neck Reconstruction*,
https://doi.org/10.1007/978-3-032-03211-9_11

- After entering level 1A, the submental artery gives off a variable number of perforators [1–4] to the platysma and overlying subdermal plexus. Perforator location may be variable, and additional information can be obtained by Dopplering the submental tissue prior to harvest.
- Venous drainage is by the submental vein, which courses parallel to the submental artery medially.
  - Submental vein may drain into the facial vein most commonly, but also may drain into the external jugular vein.
  - Care must be taken to not ligate the external jugular vein or other communicating veins in the upper neck until vascular pedicle anatomy is defined.
- Innervation to the skin is supplied by branches of V3, great auricular, and transverse cervical sensory nerves.
  - Raised as an insensate flap, with no major branches of sensory nerves dissected or included in harvest.
  - Patients are expected to have decreased sensation to the anterior neck skin after surgery.
- The marginal mandibular nerve must be identified and preserved during harvest. The nerve to mylohyoid is identified and divided in the setting of including mylohoid muscle for flap bulk.

Preoperative Care

- Obtain a thorough history of previous neck surgery or trauma that might compromise vascular pedicle integrity. History of ipsilateral comprehensive neck dissection is a contraindication. History of neck radiation, although not an absolute contraindication, should be considered in the context of flap tissue integrity and donor site closure/wound healing.
- A "pinch test" of the submental region should be performed to determined maximum flap width based on patient's individual skin laxity. Patients should be counseled to expect changes to the contour of the jawline after surgery.
- Male patients should be counseled about transfer of hair-bearing skin from the submental region to the reconstructed site. Adjuvant radiation therapy will reduce hair growth. In patients not undergoing radiation, laser hair removal therapy may be offered [3].
- A comprehensive neck exam and review of available imaging should be performed. Extensive and/or invasive level 1 lymphadenopathy is a relative contraindication. Oncologic control of occult nodal disease is possible with careful dissection of levels 1A and 1B without disruption of flap integrity or compromising oncologic outcomes [4].
- Preoperative imaging should be reviewed to help predict vascular pedicle anatomy, with particular attention to the submental venous drainage pattern, which may drain into the facial vein or, less commonly, the external jugular vein. Drainage into the external jugular vein might limit arc of rotation for medial defects.

Special Instruments and Positioning

- Helpful to use a handheld Doppler to confirm the presence of the submental artery along the underside of the mandible and perforators around the anterior belly of digastric.
- Fine dissectors are recommended to allow for careful dissection of the submental pedicle, which is often small and delicate.
- Microvascular instruments including a venous coupler are useful to have available.
- Consider suturing endotracheal tube instead of using tape to allow for wider skin prep around the chin and mandible bilaterally.

Modifications

- "Resident Modification" describes harvest of mylohyoid muscle deep to distal pedicle and perforators allowing for a safer, easier harvest [5].
- Can be harvested with vascularized bone (outer cortex of mandible).
- Can be harvested as a free flap to allow reach beyond arc of rotation of pedicle.

- Can be harvested as a "hybrid" flap with microvascular anastomosis of the facial vein and pedicled facial artery [6].
  - The facial vein is most commonly the rate-limiting factor in arc of rotation.
- Can be used as a buried flap by either raising skin off underlying adipose tissue and muscle or by de-epithelializing the flap.
  - Restoration of bulk in radical parotidectomy [7].
  - Overlay flap for salvage laryngectomy [8].
- Can be raised in a supraplatysmal plane distally to create a thinner flap and avoid injury to contralateral marginal mandibular branch of facial nerve.
- Skin island can be placed in vertical orientation in certain circumstances to improve cosmesis or in setting of prior contralateral neck surgery [9].

Pitfalls and Complications

- Risk to marginal mandibular branch of facial nerve both on ipsilateral and contralateral side.
- Loss of cervicomental angle when large flaps are harvested.
  - Can be corrected by tacking inferior skin flap to hyoid bone to restore angle.
- Overly tight closure can lead to restricted neck extension and possible wound breakdown over the mandible.
  - Consider skin grafting or placement of a wound vacuum if closure is felt to be too tight or is unable to be closed despite wide undermining.
  - Standing cutaneous deformities are common particularly along the contralateral aspect of the incision. These can be corrected after harvest or flap design can incorporate taper to minimize deformity.
  - Partial or complete flap loss is possible but rare.

Postoperative Care

- Standard incision wound care is recommended.
- Neck in a neutral or slight flexed position recommended for tight closures.
- One to two closed suction drains with removal after 3–5 days based on output.
- Flap checks as done on free flaps are unnecessary unless a hybrid flap has been performed as there is risk of venous thrombosis of a newly anastomosed vessel.

Tissue type: *Fasciocutaneous, musculocutaneous, osteomyocutaneous*
Artery: *Submental artery*
Vein: *Submental vein*
Nerve: *N/A*
Flap reach: *8 cm (but can be extended in hybrid or free flap modification). Up to the lateral canthus and zygomatic arch*
Flap size: *7 × 18 cm (but limited by ability to close donor site)*

Operative Procedure

1. Preoperative Doppler can be used to confirm the presence of submental artery and identify perforators.
2. Design skin incision in "lenticular" shape incorporated into standard neck dissection incision as indicated by ablative procedure.

   * The anterior limb of the flap is typically oriented along the inferior aspect of the mandible and not in the submental crease.
3. The skin incision is then made along anterior aspect of flap, through the platysma muscle laterally and down to mandible centrally. Subplatysmal flaps are raised superiorly to the mandible and inferiorly as indicated by ablative procedure.
4. The marginal mandibular branch of the facial nerve is identified either directly or with nerve stimulation. A fascial incision can then be made inferior to the facial nerve, allowing the nerve to be retracted superiorly and protected.

5. The facial vein is then identified proximally in its standard location posterior the submandibular gland and traced distally toward the mandible. The takeoff of the submental vein is then identified and followed distally until it approaches the anterior belly of the digastric (Fig. 11.1).
6. The submandibular gland is mobilized, and the facial artery can then be identified deep and posterior to the submandibular gland. The artery is traced toward the mandible and the submental artery identified and followed distally.

   * The submandibular gland is often removed during this step but can be left in situ depending on surgeon preference.
7. The anterior aspect of the flap can then be released from the mandible, releasing the ipsilateral anterior belly of the digastric from the mandible until the mylohyoid muscle is identified. At this point, the more distal submental pedicle and perforators can be identified.
8. Once integrity of pedicle and perforators is confirmed (helpful to use handheld Doppler at this step), the lower limb of the incision can then be completed.
9. The flap is then raised distal to proximal in a subplatysmal plane until the midline. The original submental flap as described was raised superficial to the mylohyoid muscle and requires meticulous protection of the distal pedicle and ligation of small perforators into the mylohyoid muscle.
10. Inclusion of the mylohyoid muscle, as mentioned earlier, allows for faster and safer harvest.
11. The pedicle is then mobilized as necessary to reach the surgical defect. This may require division of the distal facial vessels above the take-off of the submental vessels as well as

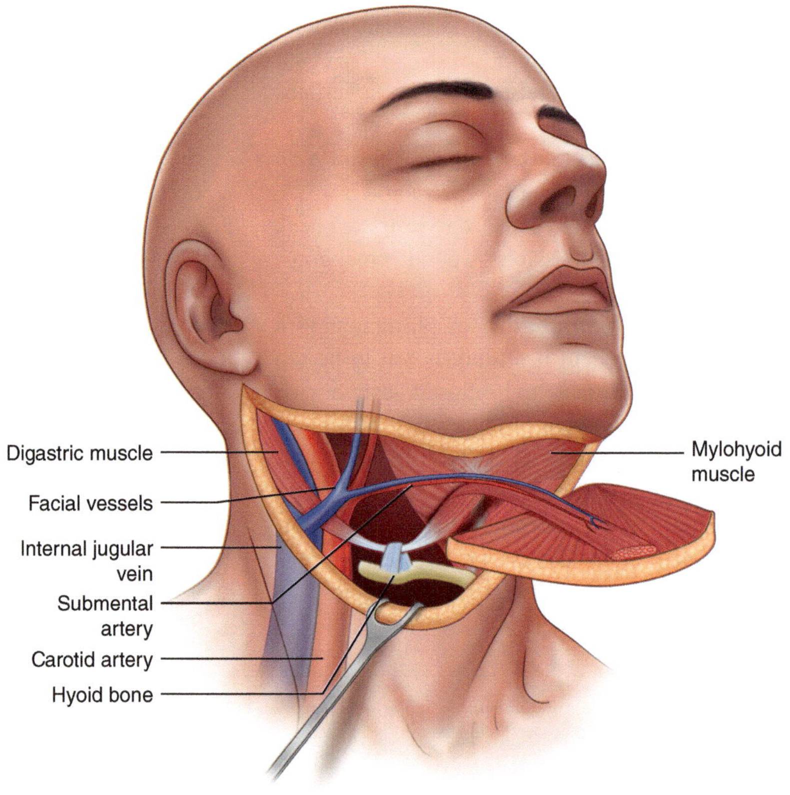

Fig. 11.1 Dissection of submental island flap pedicle demonstrating the relationship to the carotid sheath structures, digastric and mylohyoid muscles

skeletonizing of the pedicle to the external carotid and internal jugular vein.

* Additional maneuvers include a "Y–V" procedure, which divides the proximal facial vein (but requires there be a communication of the submental vein to the external jugular system), reverse flow design (division of proximal vessels with retrograde flow via angular vessels), and hybrid design [10].

12. Care is taken to position the pedicle with favorable geometry to prevent twisting or kinking that would compromise blood supply.
13. Suction drains are placed based on surgeon preference and extent of lymph node dissection performed.
14. A tension-free closure can be achieved by widely undermining the inferior skin flap in a subplatysmal plane.

* In cases requiring tracheotomy, judicious undermining is required to avoid communicating the surgical wound with the tracheotomy site.

* The cervicomental angle can be reestablished by suturing the skin flap to the soft tissues anterior to the hyoid bone.

Disclosure Statement No conflicts of interest to disclose.

References

1. Martin D, Pascal JF, Baudet J, Mondie JM, Farhat JB, Athoum A, Le Gaillard P, Peri G. The submental Island flap: a new donor site. Anatomy and clinical applications as a free or pedicled flap. Plast Reconstr Surg. 1993;92(5):867–73.
2. Faltaous AA, Yetman RJ. The submental artery flap: an anatomic study. Plasic Reconstr Surg. 1996;97(1):56–60.
3. Shields BE, Moye MS, Bayon R, Sperry SM, Wanat KA. A hairy situation: laser hair removal after Oral reconstruction. Ann Otol Rhinol Laryngol. 2018;127(3):205–8. https://doi.org/10.1177/0003489417750930.
4. Howard BE, Nagel TH, Donald CB, Hinni ML, Hayden RE. Oncologic safety of the submental flap for reconstruction in oral cavity malignancies. Otolaryngol Head Neck Surg. 2014;150(4):558–62.
5. Patel UA, Bayles SW, Hayden RE. The submental flap: a modified technique for resident training. Laryngoscope. 2007;117(1):186–9.
6. Hayden RE, Nagel TH, Donald CB. Hybrid submental flaps for reconstruction in the head and neck: part pedicled, part free. Laryngoscope. 2014;124(3):637–41.
7. Bayon R, Davis AB. Submental flap for soft tissue reconstruction following radical Parotidectomy. Otolaryngol Head Neck Surg. 2019;160(6):1130–2.
8. Hayden RE, Chang BA, Mullin DP, Patel AK, Nagel TH, Howard BE, Hinni ML, Lott DG, Donald CB. Bipedicled submental musculofascial "hammock" flap for salvage laryngectomy closure reinforcement. Head Neck. 2021;43(1):198–202.
9. Hanna TC, Gates JC, Kraus DH. Vertical Submental Island flap for head and neck reconstruction. J Oral Maxillofac Surg. 2020;78(9):1653.
10. Ferrar S, Copelli C, Bianchi B, Magri AS, Ferri A, Varazzani A, Poli T, Ferri T, Sesenna E. The submental Island flap: pedicle elongation and indications in head and neck reconstruction. J Craniomaxillofac Surg. 2014;42(6):1005–9.

Superior Labial Artery Mucosal Flap

12

Eve Tranchito, Nithin S. Peddireddy, and Cyrus C. Rabbani

History

- The superior labial artery mucosal (SLAM) flap is a variation of the facial artery myomucosal (FAMM) flap, first described by Pribaz et al. in 1992 for oral cavity and nasal reconstruction [1].

Indication and Benefits

- Reconstruction of small- to medium-sized defects of the oral cavity or nasal lining.
- Thin, well-vascularized, pliable tissue in close proximity to sites of reconstruction.
- Intraoral donor site with little cosmetic or functional deformity and morbidity.
- Can be performed as a single-stage or two-stage reconstruction.

E. Tranchito · C. C. Rabbani (✉)
Ear, Nose and Throat Institute, University Hospitals Cleveland Medical Center, Cleveland, OH, USA

Case Western Reserve University School of Medicine, Cleveland, OH, USA

Department of Otolaryngology- Head and Neck Surgery, Karmanos Cancer Center, Detroit, MI, USA
e-mail: Cyrus.Rabbani@UHhospitals.org

N. S. Peddireddy
Department of Otolaryngology- Head and Neck Surgery, Karmanos Cancer Center, Detroit, MI, USA

Anatomy

- The superior labial artery branches from the facial artery (Fig. 12.1).
  - The take-off from the facial artery is between 1 and 3.5 cm lateral to the oral commissure and is approximately 7 cm long from this point to the midline lip [2, 3].
  - Most commonly, the artery is found superior to the oral commissure; however, it can be found at the level or inferior to the commissure [4].
  - The artery typically runs in a submucosal plane between the mucosa of the upper lip and the orbicularis muscle, but variants include a largely intramuscular component.
    - Depth is at least 3 mm deep to the skin at the midpoint between the oral commissure and cupid's bow [3].
    - Can rarely bifurcate into two branches running on either side of the orbicularis muscle [5].
  - Generally, anastomoses with the contralateral superior labial artery near the upper lip midline.
  - Gives off the columellar artery once reaching the philtrum.
- Size of the flap determined by vertical height and horizontal length of upper lip mucosa.
- A cuff of orbicularis muscle is generally harvested with the mucosa.

R. Rezaee, A. Tamaki (eds.), *Local, Regional, and Free Flaps for Head and Neck Reconstruction*,
https://doi.org/10.1007/978-3-032-03211-9_12

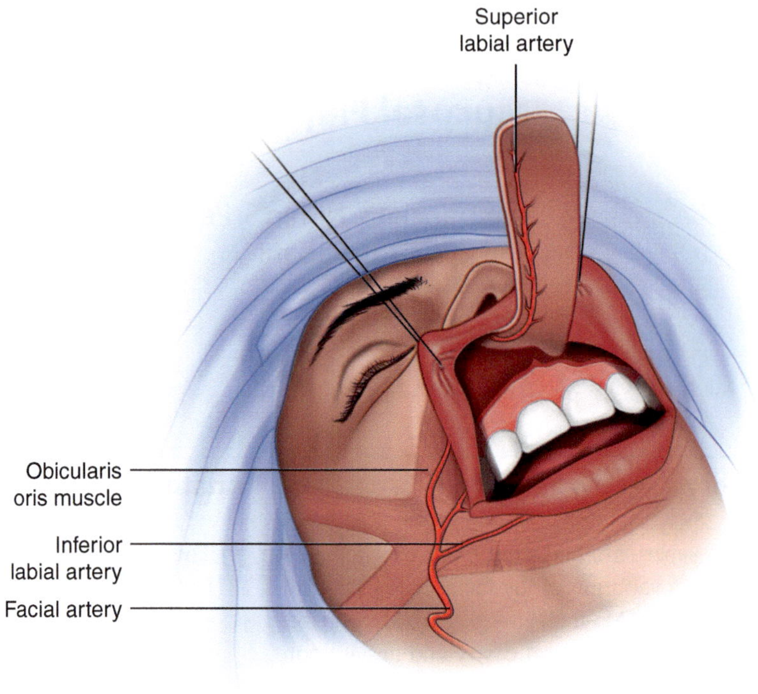

Fig. 12.1 The superior labial artery, a branch of the facial artery, supplies the superior labial artery mucosal flap. This vascular pedicle runs in the submucosal plane or intramuscular through the upper lip and/or orbicularis oris muscle

- Maintain width-to-length ratio of flap design of 5:2 for adequate perfusion [6].

Preoperative Care

- Comprehensive oral cavity examination and history to ascertain if there has been prior trauma or scars in the surrounding area that may compromise vascular anatomy or perfusion.
- Recommend smoking cessation counseling.

Special Instruments and Positioning

- Handheld Doppler is helpful to trace the vascular pedicle.
- Bite blocks and mouth retractors for visualization and improved access.
- Double prong skin hooks are useful for cheek and lip retraction.

Modifications

- Can be perfused through retrograde flow if the proximal facial artery had previously been ligated/used for other purposes such as free tissue transfer or neck dissection.
- Can include bilateral SLAM flaps for larger, complex defects, or can be incorporated with larger FAMM flaps.
- Can be raised as a bipedicled flap for complex reconstruction of the lower lip or palate.
- Can be used in conjunction with forehead flaps or free tissue transfer for complex nasal defects requiring both external and internal nasal lining.

Pitfalls and Complications

- Unilateral superior labial artery without midline anastomosis is present in up to 29% of patients [7].

- Transient donor site numbness or oronasal fistula [2].
- Risk of oral commissure or upper lip contracture at the donor site [6].
- May require a second operation for pedicle detachment.
  - Minimum time for neovascularization of 10–14 days. Commonly, pedicle maintained for 3 weeks (longer for active smokers).
  - Instruct the patient on wound care and prevent traumatic injury to the pedicle or dehiscence of the site.

Postoperative Care

- Encourage smoking cessation.
- Maintain good oral hygiene.
- Liquid or soft diet for 2 weeks.
- If the pedicle crosses intact dentition, a bite-block should be placed for approximately 10 days to protect the pedicle.

Tissue type: *Myomucosal*
Artery: *Superior labial artery*
Vein: *Concomitant vein (not necessary to identify), submucosal venous plexus*
Nerve: *None*
Pedicle length: *Variable; artery is usually incorporated into the flap but may be extended into the facial artery for more length. Average length of 50 mm²*
Flap size: *Variable based on mucosal lip height; must maintain the dry red lip, a portion of the wet red lip (≥5 mm), and a cuff of the gingival sulcus (≥5 mm)*

Operative Procedure

1. Handheld Doppler is used to identify and trace the superior labial artery on the ipsilateral side of the defect and the flap is outlined based on the trajectory of the vascular pedicle, expected arc of rotation, and size of the primary defect.
2. Inject local anesthetic.
3. The distal aspect of the flap is incised through mucosa and submucosa. Dissection proceeds until identification and ligation of the superior labial artery (Fig. 12.1).
4. Mucosa, submucosa, and possibly a small cuff of muscle may be elevated based on artery depth to the location of the facial artery takeoff.

   * It may be necessary to dissect further along the facial artery for a longer pedicle and greater transposition.
5. The flap is then transposed and inset into the defect.

   * This may require tunneling if used for nasal lining. A proximal portion of the flap within the tunnel may be demucosalized.
6. The donor site is closed primarily using absorbable sutures.

   * A second stage may be necessary at least 2 weeks later to takedown the pedicle if interpolated.

Disclosure Statement No conflicts of interest to disclose.

References

1. Pribaz J, Stephens W, Crespo L, Gifford G. A new intraoral flap: facial artery musculomucosal (FAMM) flap. Plast Reconstr Surg. 1992;90(3):421–9.
2. Momoh AO, Kelley BP, Diaz-Garcia RJ, Kulkarni AR, Kozlow JH, Bullocks JM, Lee BT. An alternative mucosal flap for nasal lining: the superior labial artery mucosal flap – an anatomic study. J Craniof Surg. 2013;24(2):626–8.
3. Sisti A, Oliver JD, Huayllani MT, Boczar D, Restrepo DJ, Nisi G, Forte AJ. Superior labial artery: anatomical considerations. Aesthet Surg J. 2019;39(7):307–8.
4. Samizadeh S, Pirayesh A, Bertossi D. Anatomical variations in the course of labial arteries: a literature review. Aesthet Surg J. 2019;39(11):1225–35.
5. Nakajima H, Imanishi N, Aiso S. Facial artery in the upper lip and nose: anatomy and a clinical application. Plast Reconstr Surg. 2002;109(3):855–6.
6. Güven E, Uğurlu AM, Başaran K, Basat SO, Yiğit B, Hafiz G, Kuvat SV. Reconstruction of intraoral defects with superior labial artery musculo-mucosal flap: a preliminary clinical study. Turk J Ear Nose Throat. 2010;20(3):118–22.
7. Magden O, Edizer M, Atabey A, Tayfur V, Ergür I. Cadaveric study of the arterial anatomy of the upper lip. Plast Reconstr Surg. 2004;114(2):355–9.

13 Supraclavicular Artery Island Flap

Emily Kamen and Urjeet Patel

History

- Mutter first described random supply cutaneous flaps from the shoulder in 1842; however, these were noted to be unpredictable with variable viability when used for head and neck reconstruction [1, 2].
- In 1979, Lamberty et al. described the supraclavicular artery as a distinct vessel able to supply a local flap in this region [3].
- Pallua et al. formally named the supraclavicular artery island flap (SCAIF) and described their methods for tunneling the flap [4, 5].
- Chiu et al. described use in detail for head and neck oncologic defects in 2009 [6].

Indications and Benefits

- Reconstruction of oral cavity, tracheostoma, pharynx, temporal bone, and cutaneous defects [7].
- Thin and pliable tissue with multiple uses.
- Supraclavicular region is often hairless.
- Minimal donor site morbidity.
- Reliable vascular anatomy with speed and ease of harvest.
- Good color and texture match for the neck [9, 10].

Anatomy

- SCAIF is an axial patterned flap based on the supraclavicular artery.
  - Most commonly a branch from the transverse cervical artery, which typically arises from the thyrocervical trunk, a branch of the subclavian artery (Fig. 13.1) [11].
    - Variation includes the supraclavicular artery arising from the suprascapular artery.
  - Found in the triangle bounded by the following:
    - Inferior: clavicle.
    - Medial: posterior border of the sternocleidomastoid muscle.
    - Lateral: external jugular vein.
  - Most commonly identified at the middle third of the clavicle.
    - Courses transversely parallel and superior to the clavicle toward the acromion, then pierces the deep fascia of the deltoid muscle [11].

E. Kamen
Department of Otolaryngology- Head and Neck Surgery, Ochsner Health, New Orleans, LA, USA

U. Patel (✉)
Department of Otolaryngology- Head and Neck Surgery, Northwestern University Feinberg School of Medicine, Chicago, IL, USA
e-mail: upatel3@cookcountyhhs.org

R. Rezaee, A. Tamaki (eds.), *Local, Regional, and Free Flaps for Head and Neck Reconstruction*,
https://doi.org/10.1007/978-3-032-03211-9_13

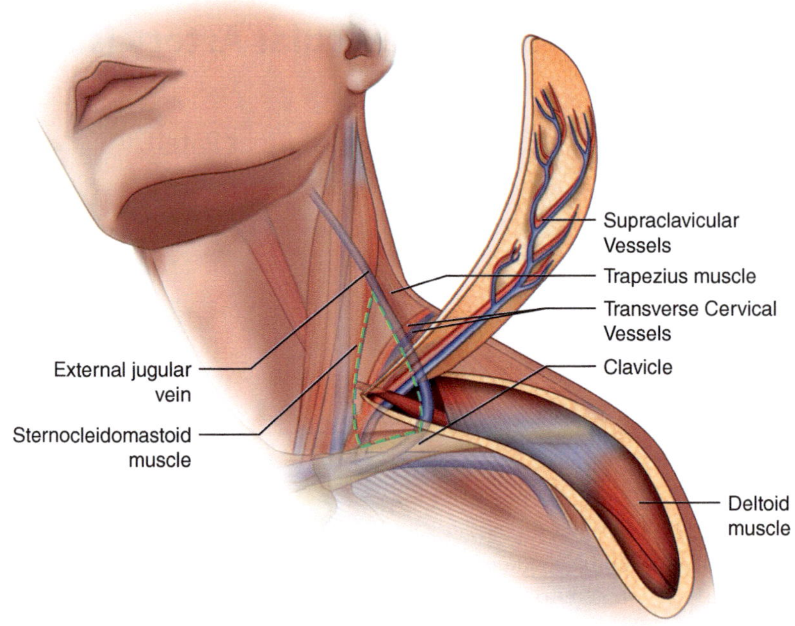

Fig. 13.1 Demonstration of supraclavicular flap and the relationship of the supraclavicular artery to triangle (green dotted line) formed by the external jugular vein, posterior border of the sternocleidomastoid muscle, and clavicle

  - Crosses the clavicle over the anterior aspect of the deltoid, generally over the lateral third of the clavicle.
  - Given the variability of the arterial supply, a bundle of tissue is generally left intact in this area during dissection rather than discrete identification and dissection of the vessel.
- Venous drainage occurs via the venae comitantes that run with the supraclavicular artery.
  - Drain via the transverse cervical vein (most commonly) and occasionally into the external jugular vein.
- Innervation to the skin is supplied by the supraclavicular nerve (from the third and fourth cervical nerves).
  - Patients may have sensation to the flap after surgery.

Preoperative Care

- Assess for history of previous neck surgery or trauma that might compromise vascular pedicle integrity. Adequate perfusion of the supraclavicular artery must be confirmed prior to proceeding.
- In the case of prior neck dissection or radiation therapy, computerized tomography (CT) angiography or duplex studies may be performed to confirm flow [11].
- Doppler ultrasound probe can be used to confirm flow of the artery in the usual anatomical location.
- History of neck radiation should be considered, although not a contraindication.

Special Instruments and Positioning

- Doppler probe can be used intraoperatively to confirm course of the supraclavicular artery.

Modifications

- This flap is generally raised as an island flap and tunneled underneath neck skin to its destination in the head and neck [7]. Alternatively, it can be raised as a peninsula and the skin of

the flap used to inset along its trajectory to its destination.
- Can be harvested as a free flap.

Pitfalls and Complications

- Maximum limit of distal skin harvest generally considered to be the deltoid tuberosity of the humerus to minimize the chance of distal flap necrosis. This generally corresponds with a length no longer than 22 cm [11].
- Dehiscence and/or cellulitis of the donor sit can occur, particularly if closed under significant tension [9, 10].

Postoperative Care

- Avoid circumferential neck ties and compression of the pedicle.
- Avoid extensive head movement or torque over the surgical site.
- One closed suction drain with removal after 3–5 days based on output.

Tissue type: *Fasciocutaneous*
Artery: *Supraclavicular artery*
Vein: *Venae comitantes*
Nerve: *Supraclavicular nerves*
Flap reach: *Zygomatic arch, temporal bone, ipsilateral floor of mouth, tonsillar fossa*
Flap size: *Skin paddle total width 6–7 cm to allow for primary closure, total length of 20–22 cm from the distal tip to the pedicle origin*

Operative Procedure

1. Doppler is used to identify the supraclavicular artery within the expected triangle. Plan a skin paddle centered around the artery tracking inferiorly along the anterolateral shoulder (Fig. 13.1).
2. Flap is raised in the subfascial plane off the deltoid muscle, with particular care as the acromion is approached to prevent injury to the pedicle. Avoid monopolar cautery on the deep surface of the flap near the acromion to minimize risk to the pedicle proximally.
3. Flap is raised anteriorly to the clavicle.
   * As a further precaution, the clavicular periosteum may be incised along its inferior edge by the pectoralis and harvested to further protect the pedicle.
4. Flap is raised posteriorly to the anterior border of the trapezius, taking care to avoid branches of the spinal accessory nerve.
   * Level V adipose and nodal tissue may be dissected if a longer arc of rotation is needed, with care to avoid excessive skeletonization of the pedicle. If done, care must be taken to not disrupt the venous drainage or proximal aspects of the external jugular vein.
5. De-epithelialize the proximal skin paddle if the flap will be tunneled.
   * If the pedicle appears to be compressed in the tunnel, consider incorporating the skin flap into the skin of the neck rather than tunneling.
6. Adequate distal perfusion of flap is confirmed prior to inset.
7. A drain is placed and the donor site is closed by widely undermining the skin to ensure a tension-free primary closure.

Disclosure Statement No conflicts of interest to disclose.

References

1. Mütter TD. Case of deformity from burns relieved by operation. Am J Med Sci. 1842;4:66.
2. Blevins PK, Luce EA. Limitations of the cervicohumeral flap in head and neck reconstruction. Plast Reconstr Surg. 1980;66(2):220–4.
3. Lamberty BG. The supra-clavicular axial patterned flap. Br J Plast Surg. 1979;32(3):207–12.
4. Pallua N, Machens HG, Rennekampff O, Becker M, Berger A. The fasciocutaneous supraclavicular artery Island flap for releasing postburn mentosternal contractures. Plast Reconstr Surg. 1997;99(7):1878–6.
5. Pallua N, Magnus NE. The tunneled supraclavicular Island flap: an optimized technique for head and neck reconstruction. Plast Reconstr Surg. 2000;105(3):842–4.

6. Chiu ES, Liu PH, Friedlander PL. Supraclavicular artery Island flap for head and neck oncologic reconstruction: indications, complications, and outcomes. Plast Reconstr Surg. 2009;124(1):115.
7. Kokot N, Mazhar K, Reder LS, Peng GL, Sinha UK. The supraclavicular artery Island flap in head and neck reconstruction: applications and limitations. JAMA Otolaryngol Head Neck Surg. 2013;139(11):1247–55.
8. Ismail H, Elshobaky A. Supraclavicular artery perforator flap in management of post-burn neck reconstruction: clinical experience. Ann Burns Fire Disasters. 2016;29(3):209–14.
9. Kozin ED, Sethi RK, Herr M, Shrime MG, Rocco JW, Lin D, et al. Comparison of perioperative outcomes between the supraclavicular Artery Island flap and Fasciocutaneous free flap. Otolaryngol Head Neck Surg. 2016;154(1):66–72.
10. Zhang S, Chen W, Cao G, Dong Z. Pedicled supraclavicular Artery Island flap versus free radial forearm flap for tongue reconstruction following Hemiglossectomy. J Craniofac Surg. 2015;26(6):527.
11. Hussaini AS, Patel UA. The submental Island pedicled flap and supraclavicular artery Island flap in a free flap practice. Plast Aesthet Res. 2022;9:30.

Temporalis Flap

14

Husain Abuhlaiqa and Sami Jean Melki

History

- First described by Golovine in 1898 for dead space obliteration following orbital exenteration.
- The technique has been refined and modified in the 1930s by Gillies who used it for facial reanimation [1–3].

Indications and Benefits

- Use in reconstruction of soft tissue defects of the scalp, forehead, orbit, cheek, nose, and oral cavity as well as in facial reanimation.
- Reliable, versatile, and relatively low risk of complications [3–6].
- Useful in cases where other reconstructive options, such as skin grafts or local flaps, are not feasible or have failed.

H. Abuhlaiqa
Otolaryngology Specialists, SEHA Clinics, Abu Dhabi, United Arab Emirates

S. J. Melki (✉)
Department of Otolaryngology- Head and Neck Surgery, American University of Beirut, Beirut, Lebanon
e-mail: sm286@aub.edu.lb

Anatomy

- The temporalis muscle is fan-shaped and arises from the lateral surface of the cranium (Fig. 14.1).
- The muscle passes medial to the zygomatic arch to insert onto the coronoid process and anterior border of the ascending ramus of the mandible.
- The muscle is innervated by the deep temporal nerves, arising from the mandibular division of the trigeminal nerve.
- The anterior and posterior deep temporal arteries are the primary blood supply, originating from the internal maxillary artery and situated on the medial aspect of the muscle [3, 4].
  - The middle temporal artery (a branch of the superficial temporal artery) anastomoses within the muscle with the deep temporal arteries.
- The muscle is covered by the superficial temporal fascia, which carries the temporal branch of the facial nerve and is continuous with the galea superiorly and the superficial muscular aponeurotic system (SMAS) inferiorly, as well as the deep temporal facia, which is continuous with the pericranium [4].
  - The deep temporal fascia is further divided into the superficial and deep layer about 2 cm superior to the zygoma.
- The temporal branch of the facial nerve crosses the zygoma about 2.4 cm anterior to the tragus [3].

R. Rezaee, A. Tamaki (eds.), *Local, Regional, and Free Flaps for Head and Neck Reconstruction*,
https://doi.org/10.1007/978-3-032-03211-9_14

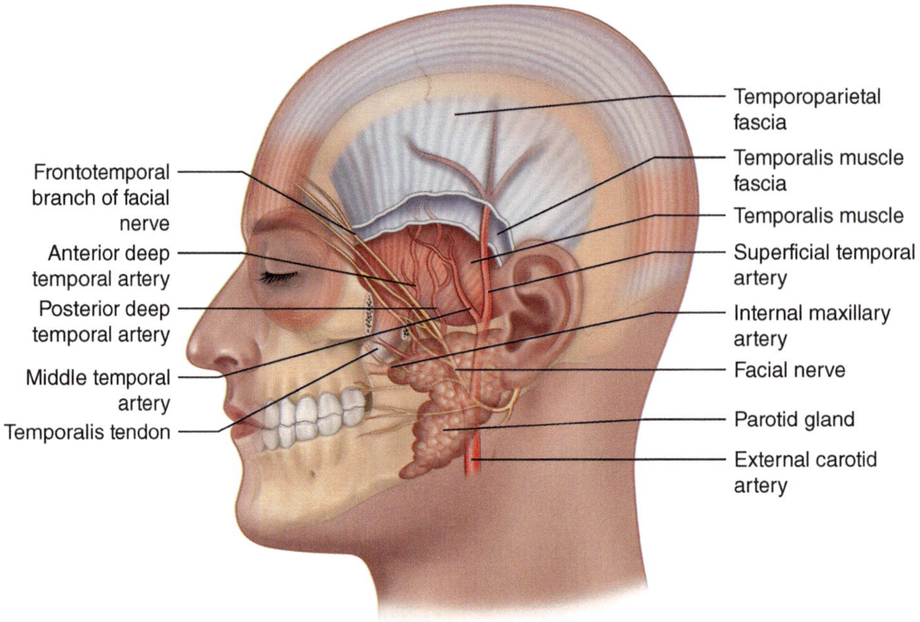

Fig. 14.1 Anatomical illustration highlighting the key vascular and neural structures associated with the temporalis muscle flap. The image shows the temporalis muscle and its fascia, including the temporoparietal and temporalis fascia. The anterior and posterior deep temporal arteries arising from the internal maxillary artery supply the temporalis flap. A segment of zygoma can be removed to increase the reach of the flap

Preoperative Care

- Obtain a thorough history, focusing on previous surgeries or embolization in the head and neck region that may affect blood supply to the flap.
- Palpate the muscle while the patient clenches their jaw to assess bulk and length of the muscle.
- Edentulous patients may have significant temporal wasting, which may make this flap inadequate.
- Use computed tomography and magnetic resonance imaging to evaluate cancer cases, ensuring tumor removal will not jeopardize blood supply to the flap.
- Document the smile type preoperatively to ensure an optimal trajectory of suspension of the muscle in cases of facial paralysis.
- Counsel the patient regarding potential cosmetic deformities, including excess bulk over the zygoma if the muscle is turned over the bone, as well as temporal hollowing.

Special Instruments and Positioning

- Optional use of a handheld Doppler to identify the temporal vessels.
- Bone saw, plates, and screws if removing a segment of zygoma is anticipated to increase the reach of the flap.
- Position supine with head turned to the opposite side of the harvest.

Modifications

- The flap can be split due to the medial and lateral blood supply.
  - The split can be performed in the coronal plane and the anterior portion is used to close the defect while the posterior portion is rotated anteriorly to prevent temporal hollowing. Alternatively, the posterior portion can be used for reconstruction and leave the anterior part intact for a better contour of the temple.

- Superiorly, parts of the pericranium can be harvested with the flap to increase length [2].
- The outer table of calvarium can be left attached to the pericranium for a limited bone graft for orbital rim or maxillary bone defects.
- Additional harvest of the tensor fascia lata and attachment to the cranial portion of the deep temporalis fascia can further lengthen the flap in facial reanimation cases [6].
- Multiple options are available to reconstruct the donor site including implants or bone cement cranioplasty [4].

Pitfalls and Complications

- Edentulous patients can have significant temporal wasting, which may preclude the use of the temporalis muscle flap [3].
- Removal of the temporalis muscle from its origin can cause temporal hollowing and facial asymmetry.
- Tumors involving the posterior wall of the maxillary sinus may put the blood supply of the flap at risk.
- Nerve injury of the frontal branches of the facial nerve or deep temporal nerves can occur during dissection, leading to weakness or paralysis of the facial muscles.
- Risk of flap failure due to vascular compromise during dissection, compression over the zygoma with sheering forces from aggressive tunneling during inset, or due to infection.
- Seroma, cosmetic deformity, and alopecia are potential minor complications [1].

Postoperative Care

- Monitor the patient for signs of hematoma or infection at the donor site.
- Physical therapy is recommended, especially in cases of facial paralysis rehabilitation.
- Speech and language pathology to review, rehabilitate, and manage swallowing difficulty and prevent associated trismus [1].
- One closed suction drain with removal after 3–5 days based on output.

Tissue type: *Myofascial*
Artery: *Anterior and posterior deep temporal arteries, middle temporal artery*
Vein: *Deep temporal veins*
Nerve: *Deep temporal branch of mandibular division of the trigeminal nerve*
Pedicle length: *8 cm of rotational radius, 135 degree arc of rotation*
Flap size: *12–16 cm diameter, with a thickness of 0.5–1.0 cm*

Operative Procedure

1. Mark incision in preauricular crease and extend superiorly into a hemicoronal incision, behind the hairline to better camouflage the incision.
   * Alternatively, a "Y" can be created at the superior most aspect of the incision for wider exposure of the muscle.
2. Dissect through skin, subcutaneous tissue, and temporoparietal fascia (TPF) until identification of deep temporalis fascia.
   * Consider infiltration with lidocaine with epinephrine for easier dissection and identification of the fascial layers [1].
3. Elevate skin flap with TPF from superior to inferior with lateral extension from the root of zygoma to lateral orbital wall.
4. Incise and elevate superficial layer of deep temporal fascia approximately 2 cm above the zygomatic arch to protect the facial nerve. Expose the zygomatic arch and elevate tissues anteriorly off bone in a subperiosteal plane. In this fashion, the frontal branch will be protected in an anatomical fashion.
5. Back elevate the skin flap posteriorly and incise edges of muscle if the entire muscle is needed for reconstruction or incise as needed after careful mapping of the vascular supply.
   * Section muscle in coronal plane if less bulk is needed.
6. Elevate the muscle off calvarial bone with a periosteal elevator and use monopolar cautery to lift firmer attachments. Preserve blood supply by remaining in the subperiosteal plane, which arises on the deep aspect of muscle and

can be visualized in the infratemporal fossa below the zygomatic arch.

7. Bluntly tunnel muscle under zygomatic arch to reach the maxilla, palate, oral cavity, or oropharynx. Place suture on deep temporalis fascia to maintain correct orientation and pass through subcutaneous tunnel. Options to increase reach:
   - Remove zygomatic arch with osteotomies if increased arc of rotation is needed and replate or wire back into place at the end of the procedure.
   - Perform a coronoidectomy to rotate muscle as an island connected by its blood supply.
   - Dissect tendinous attachments to coronoid and ascending portion of ramus off bone from transoral approach to add another centimeter of length to flap.
8. Suture flap into place with fascia facing oral cavity.
9. Close forehead with suction drain and optional pressure dressing.

Disclosure Statement No conflicts of interest to disclose.

References

1. Gillies H. Experiences with Fascia Lata Grafts in the operative treatment of facial paralysis; 1934.
2. Spanio Di Spilimbergo S, Nordera P, Mardini S, et al. Pedicled temporalis muscle flap for craniofacial reconstruction: a 35-year clinical experience with 366 flaps. Plast Reconstr Surg. 2017;139(2):468e–76e. https://doi.org/10.1097/PRS.0000000000003011.
3. Ein L, Daniyan O, Nicolli E. Temporalis muscle flap. Operat Techn Otolaryngol Head Neck Surg. 2019;30(2):120–6. https://doi.org/10.1016/j.otot.2019.04.006.
4. Smith JE, Ducic Y, Adelson R. The utility of the temporalis muscle flap for oropharyngeal, base of tongue, and nasopharyngeal reconstruction. Otolaryngol Head Neck Surg. 2005;132(3):373–80. https://doi.org/10.1016/j.otohns.2004.09.140.
5. Dallan I, Lenzi R, Sellari-Franceschini S, Tschabitscher M, Muscatello L. Temporalis myofascial flap in maxillary reconstruction: anatomical study and clinical application. J Craniofac Surg. 2009;37(2):96–101. https://doi.org/10.1016/j.jcms.2008.11.004.
6. Bajpai H, Saikrishna D. The versatility of temporalis myofascial flap in Maxillo-facial reconstruction: a clinical study. J Maxillofac Oral Surg. 2011;10(1):25–31. https://doi.org/10.1007/s12663-011-0173-5.

Temporoparietal Fascial Flap

15

Stephen Politano and Jason Thuener

History

- Introduced in 1898 by Brown and Monks, the temporoparietal fascial flap (TPFF) was used for reconstruction of the auricle [1] and eyelid [2].

Indications and Benefits

- Reconstruction of auricle, orbit, skull base, scalp, and oral cavity defects [3–6].
- Thin and pliable tissue with low donor-site morbidity.
- Option to transfer hair-bearing soft tissue with wide arc of rotation when harvested with skin.[8]
- Donor site with high likelihood of primary closure and concealed in hair-bearing scalp.
- Reliable anatomy and pedicle length [3, 7].

Anatomy

- Immediately deep to the hair follicles of the temporal scalp lies the temporoparietal fascia (TPF), which is a thin and highly vascularized layer of connective tissue (Fig. 15.1a).
- The TPF is contiguous with the superficial musculoaponeurotic system (SMAS) inferiorly and with the galea aponeurosis and occipitofrontalis superiorly.
- Layer of loose areolar connective tissue separates the TPF from the deep temporal fascia, which covers the temporalis muscle (Fig. 15.1b).
  - This avascular plane may contain crossing perforator vessels; namely from the superficial, middle, and deep temporal arteries.
- TPFF is supplied by the superficial temporal artery (STA) with a highly consistent bifurcation into frontal and parietal divisions within 0.5–2 cm anterior to the tragus and 2–3 cm above the level of the zygomatic arch [3, 7–9].
  - The STA and superficial temporal vein (STV) are the dominant vessels in the majority of patients, additional veins including the posterior auricular vein, occipital vein, and veins to the diploic space can contribute to venous drainage [3].
- Frontal branch of the facial nerve is often deep and parallels the course of the STA and STV. This branch often represents the most anterior extent of flap elevation.

S. Politano (✉) · J. Thuener
Ear, Nose and Throat Institute, University Hospitals Cleveland Medical Center, Cleveland, OH, USA

Case Western Reserve University School of Medicine, Cleveland, OH, USA
e-mail: Jason.Thuener@UHhospitals.org

R. Rezaee, A. Tamaki (eds.), *Local, Regional, and Free Flaps for Head and Neck Reconstruction*,
https://doi.org/10.1007/978-3-032-03211-9_15

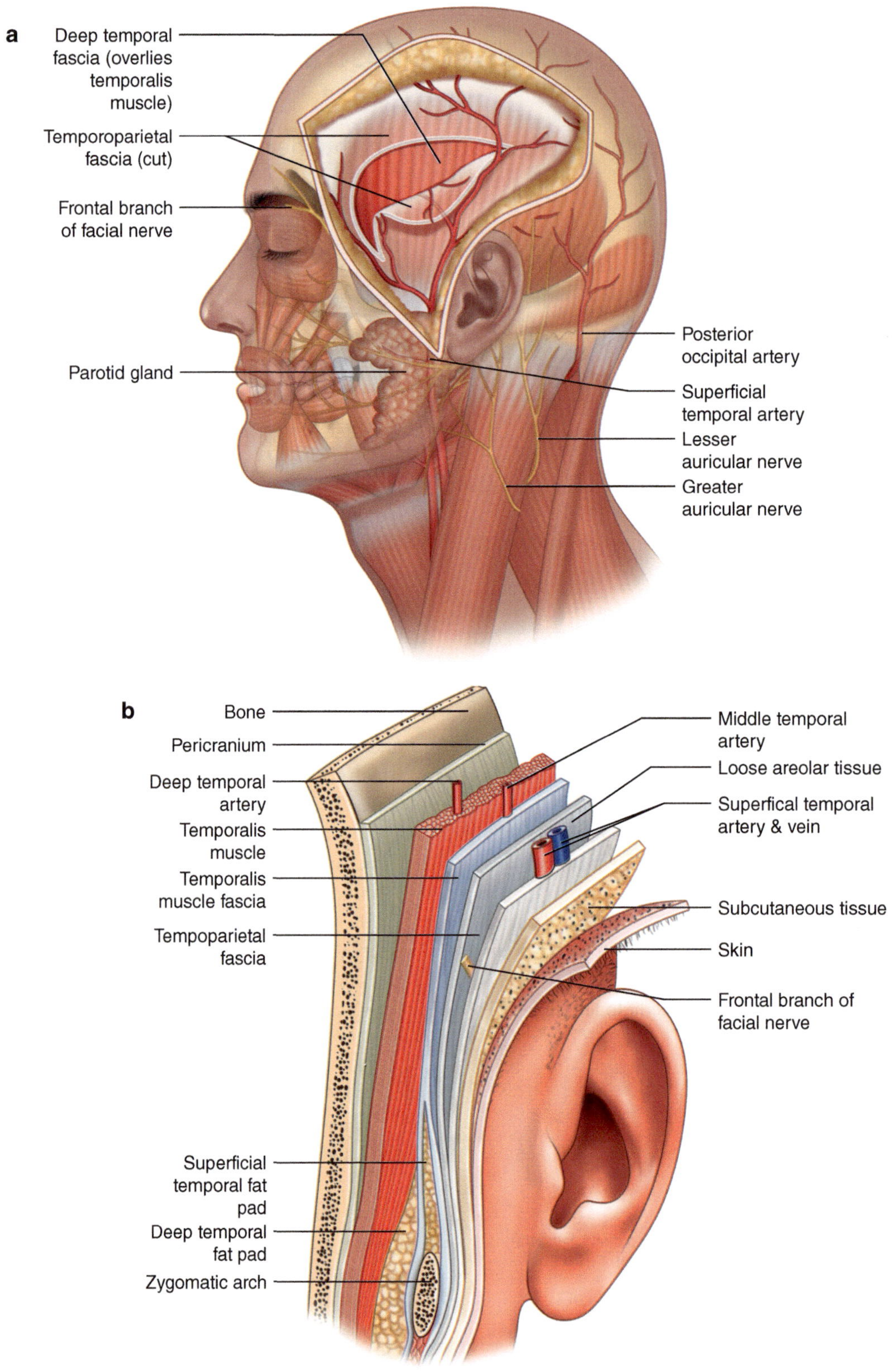

Fig. 15.1 Schematic illustration of anatomy surrounding temporoparietal fascia flap (TPFF). (**a**) General anatomical landmarks of parietal scalp and lateral face and neck. (**b**) Detailed view of layers of parietal scalp from skin to calvarium with special attention to anatomy of temporoparietal fascia, superficial temporal vessels, and frontal branch of facial nerve

- Pitanguy's line, located 0.5 cm inferior to the tragus and tangential to 1.5 cm superior and lateral to the lateral brow, is an important landmark when considering the course of the frontal branch of the facial nerve [10].
- Sensory branch of the trigeminal nerve, the auriculotemporal nerve, lies within the TPF.

Preoperative Care

- Assess skin/scalp for evidence of lesions (e.g., skin cancer) or prior trauma or surgery.
- Consideration of skin incision if including hair-bearing follicles in reconstruction.

Special Instruments and Positioning

- Preoperative marking of arterial pedicle with handheld Doppler probe.
- Position to allow for access of the entire head.
- Facelift retractors or skin hooks to aid in elevation.
- Prep and drape in sterile fashion making sure to include the expected harvest size and the orbit for consideration of monitoring the facial nerve.
- Consider shaving prior to prepping, but not a necessary step.

Modifications

- The TPFF can be used as a rotational or free flap.
- When defect is larger than expected or harvest size and additional bulk is needed, dissection can be carried deep and circumferential to the facial nerve to include more tissue.
- A chimeric two-layer TPFF can be used with inclusion of the deep temporal fascia and in some cases the temporalis muscle [3].
- The flap can be utilized mainly as a fascial flap but can incorporate skin and calvarial bone as needed [11].
- Endoscopic approach of raising the flap has been reported to minimize scarring, alopecia, and surgical time [12, 13].

Pitfalls and Complications

- Failure to meticulously dissect just deep to the hair follicles leads to hair follicle damage and subsequent alopecia.
- Vessel injury can occur since the vessels are superficial with increased tortuosity distally.
- Edema or compression on the vascular pedicle postoperatively (e.g., glasses, nasal cannula tubing).
- Nerve injury to the frontal branch of facial nerve leading to incomplete eye closure as well as possible decreased sensation secondary to loss of auriculotemporal branch of trigeminal nerve.
- Scalp hematoma.

Postoperative Care

- Avoid compression on pedicle at the temple from devices such as glasses or nasal cannula tubing.
- Frequent checks regarding the donor site skin and incision line for possible edema and presence of fluid collection.
- Consider placing surgical drain at temple.

Tissue type: *Fascial, fasciocutaneous, osteofasciocutaneous*
Artery: *Superficial temporal artery*
Vein(s): *Superficial temporal vein, posterior auricular vein, occipital vein, diploic vein*
Nerve: *Auriculotemporal nerve*
Pedicle length: *2–4 cm with the ability to be rotated into the oral cavity, mandible, midface, scalp, and auricle*
Flap size: *Approximately 14 × 17 cm without extensive scalp undermining*

Operative Procedure

1. Trace the course of the superficial temporal artery with its subsequent bifurcation into frontal and parietal divisions using a handheld Doppler probe.

2. Mark a Y- or T-shaped incision beginning in the preauricular crease and superiorly into the temporal region of the scalp.
   * The incision can bifurcate in the T or Y fashion for wider exposure of the region.
   * Consider shaving or taping hair away from desired incision line.
3. Make an incision beginning in the preauricular area through the dermis being mindful of the expected location of the vascular pedicle and branches given the superficial nature.
   * If one desires, can inject incision line with local topical anesthetic mixed with diluted epinephrine solution.
4. Elevate skin flaps just deep to the dermis being careful to avoid hair follicles and vessels (Fig. 15.1a).
   * Meticulous dissection here decreases alopecia risk.
5. Once the skin flaps are raised, the flap is elevated from the deep attachments. Begin retrograde dissection superiorly at the superior temporal line and elevate the TPF at the desired harvest size toward the pedicle inferiorly.
   * The proper plane of elevation is through the layer of loose areolar tissue separating the TPF from the muscular fascia.
6. The dissection is carried inferiorly until the expected location of the frontal branch of the facial nerve is encountered and the dissection pace should slow to allow for nerve identification and avoidance of accidental injury.
   * Handheld nerve stimulator devices can be helpful but are not required for nerve identification.
7. The vascular pedicle in the preauricular region is then freed from its remaining soft tissue attachments and ready for transfer.
   * If further length is needed for rotation, can consider dissecting the STA more inferiorly into the parotid tissue.
8. The fascial flap can be rotated into the desired recipient site under the skin.
   * At this point, can clip the pedicle vessels and use as a free flap, if desired.
9. Primary closure can be achieved with a layered closure using 3–0 Vicryl sutures for the deep dermal layers and a 5–0 Fast gut chromic for the epidermis.

Disclosure Statement No conflicts of interest to disclose.

References

1. Brown WJ. Extraordinary case of horse bite: the external ear completely bitten off and successfully replaced. Lancet. 1898;151:1533–4.
2. Monks GH. The restoration of a lower lid by a new method. N Engl J Med. 1898;139:385.
3. Horen SR, Hamidian Jahromi A, Konofaos P. Temporoparietal fascial free flap: a systematic review. Ann Plast Surg. 2021;87(6):e189–200.
4. Helman S, Kadakia S, Guthrie A, Mourad M, Mashkevich G. Temporoparietal fascia free flap for Nasoseptal perforation repair. Craniomaxillofac Trauma Reconstr. 2018;11(3):238–41.
5. Park SS, Wang TD. Temporoparietal fascial flap in auricular reconstruction. Facial Plast Surg. 1995;11(4):330–7.
6. Wurzer P, Eberl R, Kamolz LP, Parvizi D, Rappl T, Spendel S. Aesthetically and functionally satisfying reconstruction of an Achilles tendon and overlying skin defect in a 15 year old girl: a case report. Burns. 2015;41(2):e1–3.
7. Collar RM, Zopf D, Brown D, Fung K, Kim J. The versatility of the temporoparietal fascia flap in head and neck reconstruction. J Plast Reconstr Aesthet Surg. 2012;65(2):141–8.
8. Jawad BA, Raggio BS. Temporoparietal Fascia Flaps. In: *StatPearls*. Treasure Island (FL); 2022.
9. Babakurban ST, Cakmak O, Kendir S, Elhan A, Quatela VC. Temporal branch of the facial nerve and its relationship to fascial layers. Arch Facial Plast Surg. 2010;12(1):16–23.
10. Pitanguy I, Ramos AS. The frontal branch of the facial nerve: the importance of its variations in face lifting. Plast Reconstr Surg. 1966;38(4):352–6.
11. Pribaz JJ, Falco N. Nasal reconstruction with auricular microvascular transplant. Ann Plast Surg. 1993;31(4):289–97.
12. Helling ER, Okoro S, Kim G 2nd, Wang PTH. Endoscope-assisted temporoparietal fascia harvest for auricular reconstruction. Plast Reconstr Surg. 2008;121(5):1598–605.
13. Mori H, Yano T, Tanaka K, Okazaki M. Two pedicled perforator flaps combined with a fascia graft for a large lateral lumbar defect. J Plast Reconstr Aesthet Surg. 2011;64(2):274–6.

Total Lip Reconstruction: Gilles, Bernard-von Burow, and Karapandzic Flaps

16

Craig Cameron Brawley, Madeleine P. Strohl, and Evan Greenbaum

Introduction

- The lip is a common site of oncologic resection, both from oral cavity and cutaneous primary malignancies.
- There are obvious and profound functional and cosmetic roles that the lips play; reconstructive considerations after oncologic ablation strive to preserve such roles. The orbicularis oris muscle is responsible for oral competence and essential to oral intake. Reconstruction of larger lip defects should focus on maintaining such competence while minimizing aesthetic morbidity.
- Our focus is on subtotal and total lip reconstruction using three common locoregional flaps: the Gilles flap, the Bernard von-Burow flap, and the Karapandzic flap.

Anatomy

- The upper and lower lips are composed of a deep mucosal, intermediate muscular and subcutaneous, and superficial skin and vermillion layers. Layered closures and the alignment of the vermillion border is key for successful healing, function, and cosmesis.
- Oral competence is best achieved by restoring the orbicularis oris muscle sphincter during reconstruction, which must be balanced against potential microstomia.
- Arterial supply of the lips comes from the superior and inferior labial arteries, which arise from the facial arteries bilaterally.
  - Course of facial artery over mandible at antegonial notch is roughly 45 degrees toward superomedial face.
  - Distal facial artery gives off inferior labial and then superior labial branches roughly in horizontal course.
  - The inferior and superior labial branches form arcades for each lip and anastomose with the contralateral branch.
  - Arterial branches of the facial system (angular, labial) generally travel deep to the muscular layer.

C. C. Brawley
Brawley Facial Plastic Surgery, PLLC, Lansdowne, VA, USA

M. P. Strohl
Swedish Head and Neck Surgery, Swedish Medical Group, Seattle, WA, USA

E. Greenbaum (✉)
Division of Otolaryngology, Department of Surgery, John H. Stroger, Jr. Hospital of Cook County, Chicago, IL, USA

Department of Otolaryngology- Head and Neck Surgery, Northwestern University Feinberg School of Medicine, Chicago, IL, USA
e-mail: egreenbaum@cookcountyhhs.org

R. Rezaee, A. Tamaki (eds.), *Local, Regional, and Free Flaps for Head and Neck Reconstruction*,
https://doi.org/10.1007/978-3-032-03211-9_16

- After the labial branches take off, the facial artery becomes the angular artery, taking a somewhat more vertical course, just lateral to the melolabial fold and supero-laterally to the lateral nasal sidewall, roughly parallel with the angle of the pyriform aperture.
- Venous supply of the lip is primarily the superior and inferior labial veins, along with venae comitantes.
- Motor innervation comes from the bilateral facial nerves, which generally innervate orbicularis and facial mimetic musculature at the modiolus from their deep aspect. Sensory innervation comes from bilateral trigeminal nerves (V2 for upper lip and V3 for lower lip).

Preoperative Care

- Assess location of the lesion: upper versus lower lip, percentage of remaining lip after oncologic resection, involvement of the commissure.
- Assess laxity of surrounding soft tissue as a potential tissue reservoir for advancement.
- Assess facial creases that gain prominence with age; facial manipulation (smiling, frowning) may increase prominence for incision planning in younger patients, as may changing position (supine vs upright) [1].
- Counsel patient on microstomia and oral competence.
- Assess for history of prior local surgery, poor wound healing, or tobacco use.
- Determine current anticoagulation or antiplatelet therapy.
- Patient should be assessed for use of dentures or oral appliances, as resultant postoperative microstomia may interfere with use.

Special Instruments and Positioning

- Nasal intubation may simplify flap raising and closing but is not mandatory.
- Mark out melolabial, labiomandibular, and mental crease.
- Doppler can be used to identify the facial artery, angular artery, and labial branches; however, this is not required.
- Infiltration with local anesthesia with vasoconstricting agents is often used but is not mandatory.
- Monopolar cautery is often avoided, with bipolar cautery favored in order to minimize potential for thermal tissue damage.

Pitfalls and Complications

- Microstomia.
  - May significantly hinder use of dentures.
- Oral incompetence.
- Distortion of the oral commissure.
- Venous congestion can occur transiently.
- Wound dehiscence can occur if too much tension is placed on the suture lines.
- Lateralized (non-centered) defects can have pulled or tugged appearance of mouth from asymmetric flap advancement, especially with lower lip defects [2].
  - Non-centered defects of upper lip can lead to unnatural, non-centered, or angulated appearance of philtrum [3].
- For Gillies fan flap, there is complete loss of sensation of the lower lip as a full thickness incision is performed that goes through the neural supply of the lower lip. Sensation can return but may take many months.

Postoperative Care

- Antibiotics may be considered postoperatively.
  - Anti-staphylococcal coverage is appropriate if buccal mucosa is not incised and reapproximated.
  - Broader coverage may be implemented if intraoral buccal incisions and re-approximation are warranted.
- No dietary restrictions if intraoral incisions are not utilized.
  - May consider clear liquid diet (24–72 h) if buccal incisions made.

- Chlorhexidine can be used for 1 week.
- Topical petrolatum ointment (+/− antibiotic component) for cutaneous incisions.
- Avoidance of sun and rigid application of sunscreen for 4–6 months postoperatively.

I. Gillies Fan Flap

History

- The Gillies fan flap was first described by Harold Gillies in the 1920s for repair of lower lip defects [4]. Gillies was one of the founding fathers of modern plastic surgery. He made great contributions to the field through developing advanced surgical techniques to reconstruct veterans injured in World War I.

Indications and Benefits

- Reconstruction of lower lip defects between one-third and near total defects.
- Reconstruction can be done in one stage.
- Gillies fan flaps have largely fallen out of favor in its use due to denervation of the lip from the incisions required to mobilize the flap.

Modifications

- The McGregor modification is used when the vermillion of the lower lip has been removed [5]. The flap is then designed as a rectangle and can be used to reconstruct the total lower lip. The vermillion is then reconstructed using a second flap, such as a tongue flap or buccal/mucosal advancement flap.

Tissue type: *Myocutaneous*
Artery: *Bilateral superior labial arteries arising from the facial arteries*
Vein: *Bilateral superior labial veins*
Nerve: *N/A*
Flap reach: *5–7 cm (unilaterally or bilaterally)*
Flap size: *6 cm*

Operative Procedure

1. Mark the patient's melolabial crease. Mark out the size of the expected defect. The flap is designed taking into account the size of the final defect. The inferior incision is an extension of the inferior aspect of the defect. This is carried up laterally to the oral commissure, and then extends superiorly along the melolabial crease. A backcut is then performed superiorly toward the oral commissure at a 60-degree angle from the craniocaudally oriented incision. This maintains the pedicle of the superior labial artery (Fig. 16.1).
2. Incision lines are injected with lidocaine with epinephrine.
3. Incision is made through the skin and carried down full thickness through the lip, subcutaneous tissue, muscle, and mucosa.

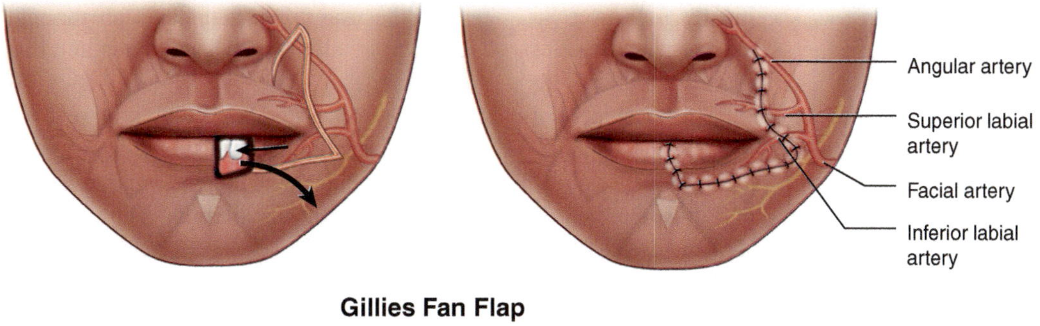

Fig. 16.1 Depiction of lip reconstruction with the Gillies fan flap

4. The leading edge is then rotated medially, pivoting around the oral commissure.
5. The vermillion border should be realigned carefully. Reestablish continuity of the orbicularis muscle.
6. Mulitlayer closure of the lip is then performed.

II. Bernard-von Burow Flap

History

- First introduced in the literature by Bernard in 1852 [6] and von Burow in 1855 [7], then Webster et al. in 1960 [8].

Indications and Benefits

- Reconstruction of total and subtotal defects of the lip.
- Applicable to both upper and lower lips.
- Benefits include local, matching tissue with similar thickness, pigmentation, and hair bearing nature, if applicable.
- No disruption or steal from the uninvolved lip.
- Better overall oral competency than free flap.
- Can be performed as outpatient surgery not requiring hospital stay.

Modifications

- There have been several modifications to this technique, with the most notable occurring in 1960 by Webster et al. [8]:
  - This technique, specifically for lower lip reconstruction, preserves mental aesthetics and sensation. The modification allows for more horizontally oriented advancement of the lip [9]. It implements four subcutaneously excised curvilinear triangles to aid in advancement: the superior two including the melolabial folds and the inferior two including the melomental folds.
- The Johanson flap was described in 1974 as another type of lower lip advancement flap, utilizing bilateral stairstep formations originating from the labiomental crease, with a subsequent excision of squares formed by the steps to allow for medial advancement [10].
  - This was further modified in 2011 to the Fernandes flap, replacing these stairstep formations with semilunar excisions for improved aesthetics [11]. Neither of these flaps utilize excised melolabial triangles for advancement, and they only alter the lower lip.

Tissue type: *Myocutaneous, mucocutaneous*
Artery: *Bilateral superior or inferior labial arteries arising from the facial arteries*
Vein: *Bilateral superior or inferior labial veins*
Nerve: *Motor innervation from facial nerve, sensory innervation from trigeminal nerve (V2 and V3 branches)*
Flap reach: *4–6 cm bilaterally*
Flap size: *5 cm bilaterally*

Operative Procedure

Upper Lip Reconstruction

1. Careful markings are made before any excisions are performed. A trapezoidal marking is made around the ablated lip superiorly toward the nasolabial angle. Four Burow triangles are also marked out, with the base of the two smaller triangles extending laterally from the superior border of the trapezoidal marking. These triangles are oriented superiorly and are situated lateral to the nose without disrupting the alar facial sulcus. The base of the two larger inferior triangles extend laterally from the oral commissure and are oriented inferiorly along the melomental folds (Fig. 16.2).
2. Incision lines are injected with lidocaine with epinephrine.
3. Using a scalpel, a full thickness excision is performed at the trapezoidal lip marking. Thereafter, the four Burow triangles are excised to the depth of subcutaneous fat to allow for bilateral advancement. The advancement flaps and lateral aspects of the Burow triangles are undermined to facilitate this.

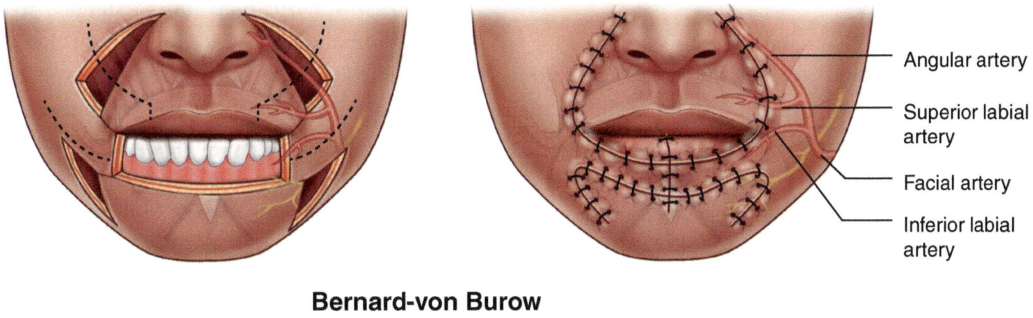

Fig. 16.2 Depiction of lower lip reconstruction with the Bernard-von Burow flap

4. The advancement flaps are closed in layers. The Burow triangles are closed primarily in layers. Anterior mucosal advancement flaps are performed if needed to restore a vermillion.

Lower Lip Reconstruction

1. Careful markings are made before any excisions are performed. A triangular marking is made around the ablated lip, oriented inferiorly toward the mentum. Two smaller Burow triangles are also marked out and oriented superiorly, with the base of these triangles extending laterally from the oral commissure (Fig. 16.2).
2. Incision lines are injected with lidocaine with epinephrine.
3. Using a scalpel and monopolar cautery, a full thickness excision is performed at the triangular lip marking. Thereafter, the two Burow triangles are excised to the depth of subcutaneous fat to allow for bilateral advancement. The advancement flaps and lateral aspects of the Burow triangles are undermined to facilitate this.
4. The advancement flaps are aligned together and closed primarily in layers. The Burow triangles are closed primarily in layers. Anterior mucosal advancement flaps are performed if needed to restore a vermillion.

III. Karapandzic Flap

History

- First introduced by Karapandzic in 1974 [12]. This is considered a modification of the Gillies fan flap.

Indications and Benefits

- Primarily used for lower lip reconstruction, although may be used for upper lip reconstruction.
- Generally useful for larger defects, up to roughly three-quarters of lip.
  - Can be used for smaller defects; however, these are often amenable to other means of locoregional closure.
- Method of elevation and flap design allows for preservation of orbicularis oris fibers and its neurovascular inputs, which in turn preserves oral competence and sensation.
- Flap design utilizes the natural facial creases that arise around the lip.
  - Incisions are thus hidden in natural creases, affording excellent aesthetic results.
- May be combined with other cheek flaps for ablative defects extending beyond the boundaries of the lip [13].

Modifications

- Variations include revised flap design at melolabial crease with more vertical component, which functions as a bilobed flap, avoiding need for extension into nasal sill.

Tissue type: *Cutaneous, myocutaneous*
Artery: *Bilateral superior or inferior labial arteries arising from the facial arteries with potential contribution from angular artery*
Vein: *Bilateral superior or inferior labial veins*
Nerve: *Motor innervation from facial nerve, sensory innervation from trigeminal nerve (V2 and V3 branches)*
Flap reach: *Circumferential advancement within confines of melolabial, labiomandibular, and mental crease*
Flap size: *Within same confines as above, predicated upon defect requirements usually up to three-quarters of lip size*

Operative Procedure

1. Mark out melolabial, labiomandibular, and mental crease (Fig. 16.3).
2. Incision lines are injected with lidocaine with epinephrine.
3. Skin incised sharply at melolabial folds, extended into a portion of the labiomandibular fold.

   * Make certain the width of the flap is proper as this will represent the height of the reconstructed segment of lip.

   (a) *For upper lip*: Incision is extended from melolabial fold into the alar base, nasal sill, and columellar base.

   (b) *For lower lip*: Incision is extended from labiomandibular fold into mental crease.
4. Incision proceeds from skin through subcutaneous fat, down to orbicularis and muscles of facial expression, which coalesce at modiolus.

   * Subcutaneous dissection undertaken bluntly with care and attention to identification and preservation of arterial branches and both sensory (trigeminal) and motor (facial) nerve branches.
5. Advancement of each raised skin flap may be examined for defect closure in a tension-free manner.

   (a) For smaller defects, the buccal layer may not warrant any treatment.

   (b) For larger defects, mucosal incisions may be required to facilitate advancement and closure.

   (c) For central defects, each flap should be advanced symmetrically; however, lateral defects may require asymmetric advancement to minimize a puckered-lip or other asymmetric appearance to the final outcome [14].
6. Vermilion is reapproximated.

   * Reapproximate the mucosal and muscular layers followed by the cutaneous layer, taking note of the alignment of the vermillion border.

   * If ablative requirements warrant sacrifice of component of orbicularis oris, the remaining muscle fibers may be opposed and sutured.
7. Mucosa reapproximated with absorbable suture.
8. Cutaneous layer reapproximated in layers.

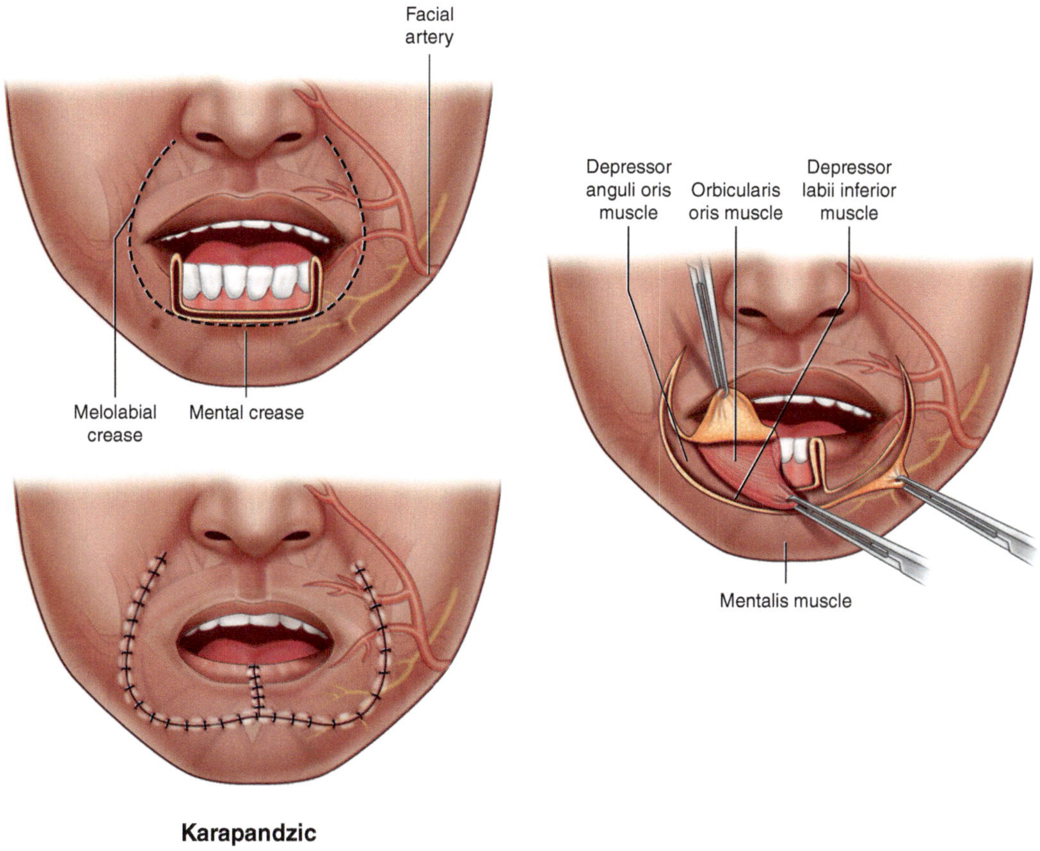

Fig. 16.3 Depiction of lip reconstruction with the Karapandzic flap

Disclosure Statement No conflicts of interest to disclose.

References

1. Gillies H, Millard DR. The principles and art of plastic surgery. Butterworth; 1957.
2. McGregor IA. Reconstruction of the lower lip. Br J Plast Surg. 1983;36(1):40–7.
3. Bernard C. Cancer de la levre inferieure: restauratio a l'aide de lembeaux quadrilataires-lateraux querison. Scalpel. 1852;5:162–4.
4. Burow CAv. Beschreibung einer neuen transplantations-methode (method der seitlichen dreiecke) sum wiederersatz verlorengegangener teile des gesichts. Berlin: Nauck; 1855.
5. Webster RC, Coffey RJ, Kelleher RE. Total and partial reconstruction of the lower lip with innervated musclebearing flaps. Plast Reconstr Surg Transplant Bull. 1960;25:360–71. https://doi.org/10.1097/00006534-196004000-00007.
6. Baker SR. Local flaps in facial reconstruction. In: Reconstruction of the scalp. Third edition. ed. Philadelphia: Elsevier/Saunders; 2014.
7. Johanson B, Aspelund E, Breine U, Holmström H. Surgical treatment of non-traumatic lower lip lesions with special reference to the step technique. A follow-up on 149 patients. Scand J Plast Reconstr Surg. 1974;8(3):232–40. https://doi.org/10.3109/02844317409084399.
8. Pirgousis P, Fernandes R. Reconstruction of subtotal defects of the lower lip: a review of current techniques and a proposed modification. J Oral Maxillofac Surg. 2011;69(1):295–9. https://doi.org/10.1016/j.joms.2010.05.079.
9. Karapandzic M. Reconstruction of lip defects by local arterial flaps. Br J Plast Surg. 1974;27(1):93–7.

10. Baker SR. Local flaps in facial reconstruction. In: Reconstruction of the lip. 2nd ed. Philadelphia: Mosby Elsevier; 2007.
11. Ong WC, Lim J, Lim TC. A modification of the bilobed and Karapandzic flap used for reconstruction of the lower lip. Plast Reconstr Surg. 2005 Jun;115(7):2154–5. https://doi.org/10.1097/01.prs.0000143916.30314.af.
12. Jackson IT. Local flaps in head and neck reconstruction. 2nd ed. St. Louis: Quality Medical Publishing; 2007.
13. Miller LE, Greene JJ. The Karapandzic flap. Operat Tech Otolaryngol. 2020;31:21–5. https://doi.org/10.1016/j.otot.2019.12.006.
14. Papel ID, et al. Facial plastic and reconstructive surgery. 3rd ed. Lip reconstruction. New York: Thieme; 2009.

Part II

Free Flap

17 Anterolateral Thigh Free Flap

Malek H. Bouzaher and Michael Fritz

History

- Initially described in the literature by Song et al. in 1984 [1].
- Popularized in the 1990s by Koshima et al. and Kimata for use in head and neck reconstruction.

Indications and Benefits

- Broad utility in reconstruction of oral cavity, oropharyngeal, pharyngeal, laryngeal, cutaneous, orbital, and skull base defects.
  - Can be used for tubed laryngopharyngectomy defects.
  - Adipofascial or fascial flap provides highly vascular thin tissue, which can be used for mucosal coverage in contracture tolerant areas (e.g., hard palate, mandibular surface reconstruction) or contour correction with long-term volume control.
  - Allows for harvest of vascularized skin, fascia, and muscle with independently mobile components.
- Harvest site provides nerve (motor nerve to vastus lateralis or lateral femoral cutaneous sensory nerve), fascia (fascia lata), and skin graft sources.
- Minimal donor site morbidity.
  - No difference in pain, cosmesis, or lower extremity function when compared to upper thigh split thickness skin graft [2].
- Generally consistent and reliable vascular anatomy with few exceptions.
  - 90% of perforators arise from descending branch of lateral circumflex system (10% from transverse branch).
  - Vascular pedicle can vary in length from 8 cm to greater than 15 cm depending on anatomy and number of perforators incorporated.
  - Arterial diameter consistently greater than 2 mm, at least one venae comitante greater than 2.5 mm [4].

Anatomy

- Lower extremity arterial supply derives from the common femoral artery, which gives off the profunda femoris, the main arterial supply to the posterolateral thigh.
- Profunda femoris gives off the lateral circumflex artery as one of its most proximal branches, from which emanates the ascending, transverse, and descending branches (Fig. 17.1).

M. H. Bouzaher · M. Fritz (✉)
Department of Otolaryngology- Head and Neck Surgery, Head and Neck Institute, Cleveland Clinic, Cleveland, OH, USA
e-mail: fritzm1@ccf.org

R. Rezaee, A. Tamaki (eds.), *Local, Regional, and Free Flaps for Head and Neck Reconstruction*,
https://doi.org/10.1007/978-3-032-03211-9_17

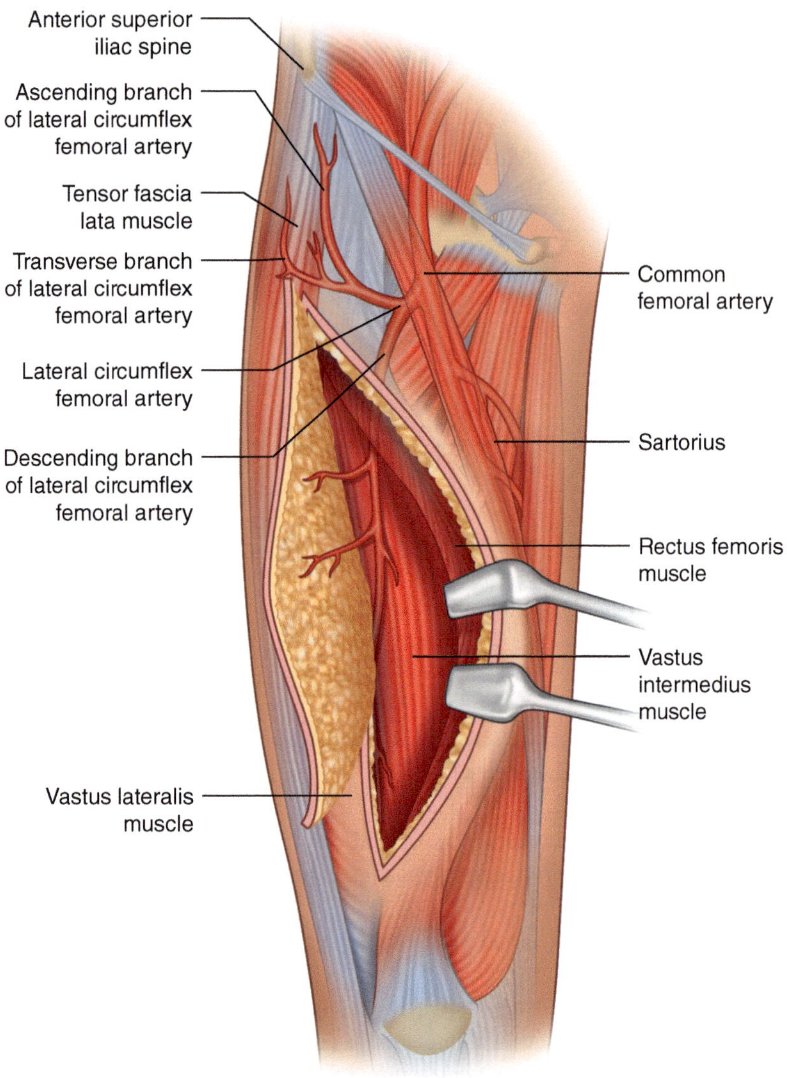

Fig. 17.1 The anterolateral thigh free flap derives its blood supply from the descending branch of the lateral circumflex femoral artery. The rectus femoris muscle is retracted medially showing the artery running between the rectus femoris and vastus lateralis muscles in the anterior compartment of the thigh. Perforators may be myocutaneous, travelling through the vastus lateralis muscle, or septocutaneous, travelling through the intermuscular septum. Myocutaneous perforators require dissection through the vastus lateral muscle in perforator-based flaps

- The lateral circumflex artery provides branches to the rectus femoris proximally.
- The descending branch of the lateral circumflex artery travels between the rectus femoris and vastus lateralis muscles in the anterior compartment of the thigh.
- Cutaneous perforators may come from the descending branch (90%) or transverse branch (10%) of the lateral circumflex artery.
- Perforators may be myocutaneous (~87%), travelling through the vastus lateralis muscle, or septocutaneous (~13%), travelling through the intermuscular septum [5].
  - Type I myocutaneous perforators emanate from the descending branch of the lateral circumflex artery and have a relatively short course (2–3 cm) through the vastus lateralis muscle traveling in a medial-to-lateral direction.
  - Type II myocutaneous perforators emanate from the transverse branch of the lateral circumflex artery and have a prolonged course (up to 10 cm) through the vastus lateralis muscle traveling in a superior to inferior direction [6].
- Venous drainage is from accompanying venae comitantes, which have variable branching and patterns of communication.

- Very rarely, the dominant perforator system flows directly across the rectus femoris from the profunda artery.
- Innervation is supplied by the lateral femoral cutaneous nerve, which supplies sensation to the anterolateral thigh, and travels in the deep subcutaneous (suprafascial) plane [7].

Preoperative Care

- Preoperative decision and protection of surgical leg.
  - Generally left selected (more rapid return to driving). Other patient factors may be considered in site selection, for example in equestrians, right-handed bowlers, and commercial truck drivers (manual transmission).
- Assess for history or scars from prior surgery or trauma that may compromise vascular anatomy or perfusion to the skin.
- Donor thigh tends to be thicker proximally and thinner distally.

Special Instruments and Positioning

- Thigh is positioned to allow for easy access to mid-thigh and lateral intermuscular septum.
- Perforators localized with Doppler probe near mid-point between anterior superior iliac spine (ASIS) and superolateral patella [8].
  - This facilitates incision position and design, particularly when a smaller incision is desired.
- No special equipment or tourniquet necessary for harvest.
- Some surgeons may consider light bump under hip for some patients based on body habitus.

Modifications

- Flap utility is vastly amplified when harvested as a perforator flap; provides significantly longer pedicle reach and eliminates muscle bulk.
- Perforators can be followed distally to subdermal region to allow for aggressive thinning of subcutaneous fat to adapt a thicker thigh for mucosal reconstruction.
- Skin paddle and subcutaneous fat can be removed to create a very thin and highly vascularized fascia lata flap, which has utility in multiple settings (e.g., palate, orbital, rescue flap for osteoradionecrosis, total and complex nasal reconstruction) [9].
- Flaps may be split and modified on multiple perforators; a separate muscular paddle can be harvested on distal descending circumflex system (e.g., skull base reconstruction).
- Perforator dissection can be done without performing the lateral incision, allowing for the majority of flap harvest to take place without committing to size or shape prior to completion of the resection.

Pitfalls and Complications

- Variable perforator anatomy and intramuscular course requires exposure and preservation along entire course to prevent injury and flap compromise.
- Excess bulk on vascular pedicle (if perforator dissection not employed) limits flap reach and utility.
- Failure to preserve at least one nutrient branch to the rectus femoris from the lateral femoral circumflex artery may result in ischemic necrosis of the muscle.
- Aggressive undermining to achieve closure can result in cutaneous compromise and skin necrosis.
  - In circumstances of wider flap harvest and challenges with primary donor site closure, wound vacuum and/or split thickness skin grafting can be utilized.

Postoperative Care

- One to two closed suction drains, usually removed within 7–14 days based on output [3].
- Patient is encouraged to mobilize as soon as possible, with no limitations on ambulation.

Tissue type: *Myocutaneous, adipofascial, fasciocutaneous*
Artery: *Descending or transverse branch of lateral circumflex artery*
Vein: *Venae comitantes*
Nerve: *Lateral femoral cutaneous nerve (motor), lateral femoral cutaneous nerve (sensory)*
Pedicle length: *10–16 cm, however, can be longer depending on whether distal perforators are used*
Flap size: *Maximum reported 40 × 15 cm*

Operative Procedure

1. A line is drawn from the ASIS to the superolateral border of the patella; this approximates the location of the intermuscular septum separating the rectus femoris and vastus lateralis muscles.

   * Handheld Doppler probes may be used to ascertain the approximate location of the cutaneous perforators, which are typically within 3–5 cm of the midpoint of this line.
2. A straight-line medial skin incision is designed over the approximate location of the mid portion of the rectus femoris muscle.

   * Elliptical incisions at onset are avoided as this limits the ability to adapt flap design to perforator location once located.
3. Dissection is carried down through skin, subcutaneous fat, and fascia and the rectus femoris muscle is identified.

   * Care should be taken to ensure that the incision is not placed too laterally as this may result in inadvertent transection of perforators as they reach the skin.

   * Placement of the incision too medially may result in difficulty achieving primary closure.
4. The fascia overlying the rectus femoris is then incised and the muscle belly retracted medially.
5. The pedicle (descending branch of the lateral circumflex artery and two vena comitantes) is then identified running between the rectus femoris and vastus lateralis on top of the vastus intermedius muscle (Fig. 17.1).
6. Perforators are identified in the intermuscular septum (septocutaneous) or superficial to the vastus lateralis (myocutaneous) as they enter the fascia lata and travel toward the skin.

   * If perforators are not immediately identifiable, dissection should continue superiorly and inferiorly until they are visualized.
7. Attention is turned to isolation of the vascular pedicle, which is done by making an incision in the fascia adjacent to the pedicle over the nerve to the vastus lateralis.

   * The pedicle is then traced proximally until sufficient length is exposed.

   * If only a single branch to the rectus femoris is identified, this should serve as a stopping point for dissection.

   * Branching and/or communication between vena comitantes may occur at any point along the length of the pedicle.
8. The flap can be harvested with various amounts of the vastus lateralis muscle or can be harvested as perforator based. Perforators can be carefully dissected from distal to proximal until they join the vascular pedicle. As they are often myocutaneous, muscle fibers of the vastus lateralis must be transected to trace the course of the perforators.
9. With the perforator course and entry points well-defined, a lateral skin incision is designed based on the defect.

   * This design is typically elliptical, or an M-plasty (removal of standing cutaneous deformities from the end of a linear wound) can be employed proximally or distally to capture increased flap width around perforators.

   * Incision is initially carried down to but not through the fascia lata.
10. The fascia lata is then incised with care to avoid injury to the previously dissected perforators. Additional vascularized fascia may be included to provide further reconstructive substrate for defect coverage or contour.
11. With the flap now isolated on perforators from their exit point from the vastus lateralis to their entry into the main pedicle, these vessels are now freed circumferentially

through the muscle with near complete sparing of the muscle.

* Hemostasis is maintained with aggressive use of clips for branching vessels and careful use of electrocautery or other hemostatic dissection devices.

12. After vessels are completely isolated to their entry into the vascular pedicle, the distal continuation of the descending pedicle is isolated and divided.

    * The pedicle is now free proximally until the takeoff of the major nutrient vessel to rectus femoris and individual vessels are isolated.

    * Adjacent branches of motor nerve to vastus lateralis are spared as they are freed from the pedicle.

    * Notably, if the ablative defect is yet undefined, all perforator and pedicle dissection can be performed prior to the creation of the lateral skin incision. This dissection, however, is more facile with a fully mobilized and defined flap.

13. Primary closure of a thigh defect is almost always possible.

    * Patient factors affecting closure include flap size (width), tissue laxity, density of subcutaneous tissue, skin quality.

    * If necessary to achieve primary closure, the skin and subcutaneous tissue can be undermined in a suprafascial plane taking care to avoid transection of cutaneous perforators.

    * Surgical drains should be placed deep to the rectus femoris muscle.

    * High tension closures can be supplemented with incisional wound vacuum.

    * In the rare event that advancement closure is not possible, a skin graft and overlying wound vacuum is applied to exposed muscle.

Disclosure Statement No conflicts of interest to disclose.

References

1. Song YG, Chen GZ, Song YL. The free thigh flap: a new free flap concept based on the septocutaneous artery. Br J Plast Surg. 1984;37(2):149–59.
2. Benjamin T, Zebolsky AL, Haddad AF, Ochoa E, Plonowska-Hirschfeld KA, Park AM, Seth R, Knott PD. Anterolateral thigh free flap versus thigh split thickness skin graft: comparison of morbidity in the first 30 days. Facial Plast Surg Aesthet Med. 2023;25(2):108–12.
3. Hanick A, Meleca JB, Fritz MA. Early discharge after free-tissue transfer does not increase adverse events. Am J Otolaryngol. 2020;41(2):102374.
4. Yu P. Characteristics of the anterolateral thigh flap in a Western population and its application in head and neck reconstruction. Head Neck. 2004;26(9):759–69.
5. Wei FC, Jain V, Celik N, Chen HC, Chuang DC, Lin CH. Have we found an ideal soft-tissue flap? An experience with 672 anterolateral thigh flaps. Plast Reconstr Surg. 2002;109(7):2219–26. discussion 2227-30
6. Shieh SJ, Chiu HY, Yu JC, Pan SC, Tsai ST, Shen CL. Free anterolateral thigh flap for reconstruction of head and neck defects following cancer ablation. Plast Reconstr Surg. 2000;105(7):2349–57. discussion 2358-60
7. Yu P. Reinnervated anterolateral thigh flap for tongue reconstruction. Head Neck. 2004;26:1038–44.
8. Landuyt KV. The anterolateral thigh flap for lower extremity reconstruction. Semin Plast Surg. 2006;20(2):127–32.
9. Arianpour K, Meleca JB, Liu SW, et al. Evaluation of anterolateral thigh fascia Lata rescue flap for mandibular osteoradionecrosis. JAMA Otolaryngol Head Neck Surg. 2023;

18 Fibular Free Flap

Kate Clancy and Nicole Fowler

History

- Use of a vascularized fibular bone flap dates back to 1975, as described by Taylor; however, it was Hidalgo in 1989 who first described the use of the fibula for repair of segmental mandibulectomy defects in the head and neck [1, 2].

Indications and Benefits

- Due to the large amount of available bone, the fibula is an ideal donor site for large segmental defects with the need for multiple osteotomies, especially subtotal or total mandibulectomy defects. The fibula can also be utilized in maxillary/midface reconstruction [1, 3, 4].
- Thick bone stock allows for the placement of dental implants.
- Associated skin paddle is thin and pliable.
- Flap is easily raised simultaneously (two-team approach).

Anatomy

- The fibula is a limited weight-bearing bone that functions to stabilize the knee and ankle joints.
- The bone has a triangular shape, where the peroneal artery runs along the medial surface. Plating is performed on the lateral surface, and the septum containing perforators attaches to the posterior surface.
- The popliteal artery bifurcates into the anterior and posterior tibial arteries, and the peroneal artery branches from the posterior tibial 2–3 cm distal to this bifurcation. The peroneal artery supplies septocutaneous perforators to the skin as well as the periosteal blood supply to the bone. The artery and associated venae comitantes remain in close proximity to the medial surface of the fibula bone as it descends distally in the leg and runs between the tibialis posterior and flexor hallucis longus muscles (Fig. 18.1) [1].

K. Clancy
Ear, Nose and Throat Institute, University Hospitals Cleveland Medical Center, Cleveland, OH, USA

Case Western Reserve University School of Medicine, Cleveland, OH, USA

Mercy Health Lorain Hospital, Lorain, OH, USA

N. Fowler (✉)
Department of Otolaryngology- Head and Neck Surgery, University of Virginia Health, Charlottesville, VA, USA
e-mail: EJZ6PH@uvahealth.org

R. Rezaee, A. Tamaki (eds.), *Local, Regional, and Free Flaps for Head and Neck Reconstruction*,
https://doi.org/10.1007/978-3-032-03211-9_18

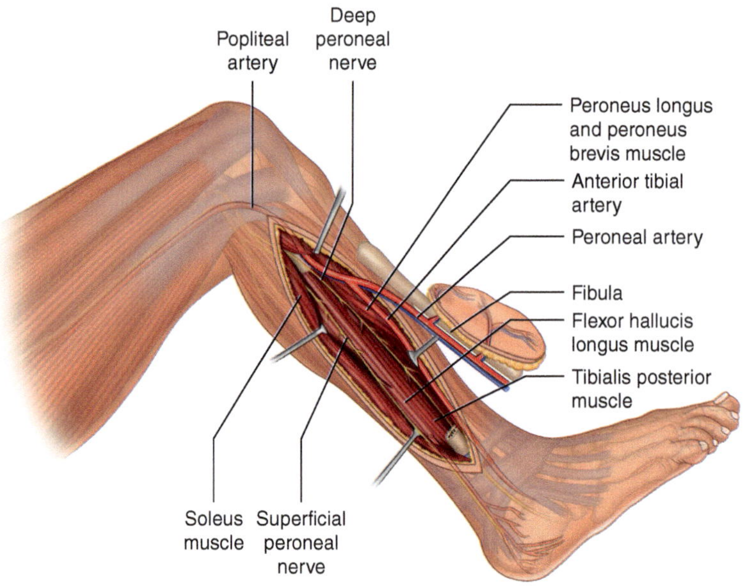

Fig. 18.1 Fibula osteocutaneous flap pedicled on the peroneal artery and venae comitantes. The surrounding lower leg musculature remain in situ

- Peroneal artery is approximately 1.5–4 mm in diameter.
- The lower leg is divided into four muscular compartments (anterior, lateral, deep posterior, and superficial posterior). The lateral compartment overlies the fibula bone and is separated from the anterior and posterior compartments by intermuscular septa. The anterior and posterior compartments are separated by the interosseus membrane [1].
  - *Lateral compartment contents*: peroneal longus, peroneal brevis muscles. General function: foot eversion.
  - *Anterior compartment contents*: tibialis anterior, extensor hallucis longus, extensor digitorum brevis, peroneus tertius. General function: dorsiflexion.
  - *Superficial posterior compartment contents*: gastrocnemius, soleus, and plantaris muscles. General function: plantarflexion.
  - *Deep posterior compartment contents*: tibialis posterior, flexor hallucis longus, flexor digitorum longus. General function: plantarflexion.
- *Topographical landmarks*: Septocutaneous perforators supplying the skin via the posterior crural septum can be estimated at the 1/2, 2/3 and 3/4 points, 2 cm posterior to a line drawn from the fibular head superiorly and the lateral malleolus of the ankle inferiorly [9].
- Due to the higher concentration of perforators at the distal aspect of the fibula, the skin paddle should be centered over the distal and middle third of the leg [1, 9].

Preoperative Care

- History and physical exam will assist in discovering any compromised state of the lower extremities (e.g., prior surgery or trauma, history of deep vein thrombosis, or presence of peripheral vascular or cutaneous disease).
- Anterior and posterior tibial pulses can be palpated.
- Computed tomography (CT) or magnetic resonance angiography (MRA) of the lower extremities confirms patency of anterior and posterior tibial arteries (identify absence due to anatomic variation or presence of atherosclerosis). Alternatively, a vascular ultrasound of the lower extremity can be performed by appropriately trained technicians.
- *Which leg to choose?* In a setting where both legs have appropriate vasculature and a skin paddle will be used, the decision of which leg to choose depends on the desired location of the skin paddle (internal versus external) and

the location of the recipient vessels (anterior versus posterior) [1].
  - An internal (intraoral) defect can be reconstructed using:
    Contralateral leg, vessels exiting posteriorly (most common).
    Ipsilateral leg, vessels exiting anteriorly.
  - An external (cutaneous) defect can be reconstructed using:
    Ipsilateral leg, vessels exiting posteriorly.
    Contralateral leg, vessels exiting anteriorly.
  - Special consideration to use the left leg so as not to interfere with driving.

Special Instruments and Positioning

- Use of handheld Doppler can assist with locating perforators for the skin paddle design.
- An appropriately sized thigh tourniquet (350 mmHg, <2 h).
- Leg can be propped up on foot stop, so the knee is at 90°. Alternatively, a suspension system can be used to suspend the leg.
- Tilting bed slightly to the contralateral side can be helpful to keep leg in position in certain patients whose body habitus favors external rotation at the hip prompting challenges with harvest.

Modifications

- Computer-assisted planning with custom cutting guides (mandible and fibula) can be used. This may have the benefit of decreased intraoperative time and ischemia time with similar levels of accuracy when compared to the traditional osteotomy approach [6, 7].
- Dental implants can be considered and placed at the time of initial reconstruction or in a delayed fashion.
- A double-barreled fibula flap can be used to increase the height of the reconstructed mandible or midface [8].
- Lateral sural cutaneous nerve can provide sensation to the flap, if desired [1].

Pitfalls and Complications

- Reliability of the skin paddle harvested with the fibula free flap is controversial. Increasing the length of the skin paddle may help overcome variations in perforator location.
- Mobility of the skin paddle in relation to the bone is limited compared to other bone-containing flaps. Measures can be taken to improve this skin paddle mobility in relation to the bone by releasing the septum from the bone away from the perforator, but this must be done with caution to not twist or compromise the perforator during inset.
- 4–6 cm of proximal fibula must be preserved to ensure protection of the common peroneal nerve (injury to this nerve would cause foot drop) and minimize impact on knee function.
- 6 cm of distal fibula must be preserved to avoid ankle joint instability.
- Lack of preoperative confirmation of appropriate lower extremity vasculature could lead to foot ischemia.
- Atherosclerosis of the peroneal artery could lead to difficulty in free flap vessel anastomosis.
- *Donor site morbidity*: wound dehiscence and/or skin graft loss leading to peroneal tendon exposure. Overall, function of the donor leg is reasonable and should not affect activities of daily living. However, decreases in range of motion and sensory disturbances can be seen [5].

Postoperative Care

- Foot should remain elevated postoperatively.
- If a split thickness skin graft is placed, a bolster or wound vacuum is placed and removed within 5–7 days.
- A posterior splint/cast or boot can be applied. May not need in setting of a wound vacuum or primary closure.
- One closed suction drain is used with removal after 3–5 days based on output.
- Early ambulation is possible, although controversial. Usually limit toe-touch weight bear-

ing until after 5 days. Physical therapy can be ordered to maximize recovery in those with identified postoperative mobility issues.

Tissue type: *Osseous, osteocutaneous*
Artery: *Peroneal artery*
Vein: *Venae comitante*
Nerve: *Lateral sural cutaneous nerve*
Pedicle length: *Dependent on the amount of bone being harvested. Can be increased by dissection of proximal (unused) fibula*
Flap size: *Up to 25 cm of bone can be harvested with maximum skin paddle width of 14 cm and length of 30 cm*

Operative Procedure

1. Mark the approximate location of the intramuscular septum by marking from the fibular head to the lateral epicondyle of the ankle.
   * Doppler can be used to identify perforators to the skin, which are located more distally in the leg.
   * If using a torniquet, exsanguinate the lower extremity using Esmarch wrap (or gravity) and inflate tourniquet to 350 mmHg.
2. Incise the skin at the expected anterior skin paddle border. A suprafascial dissection is performed until past the peroneus tendon.
3. Incise the fascia overlying the peroneus longus and brevis. Reflect the skin paddle posteriorly and perform gentle blunt dissection until septocutaneous perforators are identified.
   * If no septocutaneous perforators are identified, a proximal musculocutaneous perforator can be used to supply an island of skin.
   * If no perforators are identified, additional muscle could be harvested and left to granulate in the mouth.
4. Dissect peroneal muscles from fibula toward anterior compartment, leaving a few millimeters of muscle along the bone ("cobblestone appearance"), which protects the blood supply of the underlying bone.
5. Enter anterior compartment (incise anterior intermuscular septum) and raise anterior tibialis, extensor digitorum longus, and extensor hallucis longus off fibula until reaching the interosseous septum (Fig. 18.1).
   * The deep peroneal nerve, anterior tibial artery, and anterior tibial vein are identified and preserved in the anterior compartment.
6. Enter interosseous septum halfway between fibula and tibia (entering deep posterior compartment) and release up as far as possible.
   * If not done, will prevent fibula from being retracted laterally.
7. Perform osteotomies.
   (a) Ensure at least 4–6 cm of bone distal to the fibular head and 6 cm proximal to lateral malleolus are preserved.
      * The maximum amount of fibula bone is typically harvested with the option of performing additional osteotomies and discarding unwanted bone later, as this will help with visualization during pedicle dissection and increase pedicle length.
   (b) Use a right angle to dissect around fibula bone, enough to place malleable underneath the bone for protection. This is especially important proximally as the pedicle is at risk just medial to the bone.
   (c) Use saw to cut bone while your assistant irrigates to minimize thermal damage to bone.
8. Bone clamps or large bone hooks applied proximally and distally will aid in retraction.
9. Identify distal peroneal artery and venae comitantes and ligate. Trace pedicle proximally through the tibialis posterior muscle until reaching the bifurcation of the peroneal artery from the posterior tibial artery.
10. Identify the amount of bone needed for reconstruction and remove soft tissue and periosteum from the proximal bone using a large periosteal elevator, knife, or osteotome.

11. Once margins are negative (and dimensions of needed skin paddle are confirmed), posterior skin paddle back cuts can be made, dissecting through the fascia. Identify and ligate branches to soleus as the soleus muscle is dissected off, followed by dissection of flexor hallucis longus muscle. A 1 cm cuff or more of these muscles can be harvested if indicated by the defect.

    * Care must be taken not to injure the sural nerve and lesser saphenous vein along this posterior aspect.

    * Posterior skin paddle back cuts may be performed prior to the osteotomies if desired and skin paddle size is known and based on surgeon preference.
12. Ensure full dissection of pedicle to the level of the posterior tibial vascular bundle, ligate artery and vein, and bring flap to head for fixation, inset, and microvascular anastomosis.

    * If using computer-assisted planning, apply cutting guides to fibula to perform osteotomies. Custom or pre-bent plate and also dental implants can be applied and inserted while flap is still perfused, if desired.
13. Ensure hemostasis and perform closure of the donor site (primary closure or use of split thickness skin graft depending on size of the skin paddle harvested) and placement of suction drain.

Disclosure Statement No conflicts of interest to disclose.

References

1. Urken ML, Cheney ML, Blackwell KE, Harris JR, Hadlock TA, Futran N. Atlas of regional and free flaps for head and neck reconstruction: flap harvest and insetting. 2nd ed. Philadelphia: Wolters Kluwer Health – Lippincott Williams & Wilkins; 2012.
2. Hidalgo DA. Fibula free flap: a new method of mandible reconstruction. Plast Reconstr Surg. 1989;84(1):71–9. https://doi.org/10.1097/00006534-198907000-00014.
3. Genden EM. Reconstruction of the head and neck: a defect-oriented approach. Stuttgart/New York: Thieme; 2012.
4. Wei FC, Seah CS, Tsai YC, Liu SJ, Tsai MS. Fibula osteoseptocutaneous flap for reconstruction of composite mandibular defects. Plast Reconstr Surg. 1994;93(2):294–304. https://doi.org/10.1097/00006534-199402000-00009.
5. Anthony JP, Rawnsley JD, Benhaim P, Ritter EF, Sadowsky SH, Singer MI. Donor leg morbidity and function after fibula free flap mandible reconstruction. Plast Reconstr Surg. 1995;96(1):146–52. https://doi.org/10.1097/00006534-199507000-00022.
6. Barr ML, Haveles CS, Rezzadeh KS, et al. Virtual surgical planning for mandibular reconstruction with the fibula free flap: a systematic review and meta-analysis. Ann Plast Surg. 2020;84(1):117–22. https://doi.org/10.1097/SAP.0000000000002006.
7. Roser SM, Ramachandra S, Blair H, et al. The accuracy of virtual surgical planning in free fibula mandibular reconstruction: comparison of planned and final results. J Oral Maxillofac Surg. 2010;68(11):2824–32. https://doi.org/10.1016/j.joms.2010.06.177.
8. He Y, Zhang ZY, Zhu HG, Wu YQ, Fu HH. Double-barrel fibula vascularized free flap with dental rehabilitation for mandibular reconstruction. J Oral Maxillofac Surg. 2011;69(10):2663–9. https://doi.org/10.1016/j.joms.2011.02.051.
9. Yu P, Chang EI, Hanasono MM. Design of a reliable skin paddle for the fibula osteocutaneous flap: perforator anatomy revisited. Plast Reconstr Surg. 2011;128(2):440–6. https://doi.org/10.1097/PRS.0b013e31821e7058. PMID: 21502907

19 Gracilis Free Flap

Arvind Badhey and Alice L. Tang

History

- First described by Harii et al. in 1976 as a musculocutaneous flap before it was popularized for use in facial reanimation [1].

Indications and Benefits

- Myocutaneous or muscular reconstruction of soft tissue defects of the oral cavity, larynx, pharynx, cutaneous, and skull base defects as well as dynamic facial nerve reanimation [2–5].
- Thin, slender muscle, with a large well-defined and predictable motor nerve innervation.
- Consistent and reliable vascular anatomy.
- Provides ample tissue for dynamic reconstruction and excursion when reinnervated [2, 3].
- Muscle can be thinned segmentally to trim excess bulk prior to reanimation [2, 3, 5].

Anatomy

- The dominant pedicle is the terminal branch of the adductor artery, which arises either from the medial circumflex or profunda femoris artery (Fig. 19.1) [6].
- The adductor artery runs along the adductor longus anteriorly and the adductor brevis/magnus muscle posteriorly before entering the gracilis muscle belly at the junction of the upper third and lower two-thirds.
  - This point is typically 8–10 cm inferior to the pubic tubercle.
  - Branches to the adductor muscles must be ligated to obtain a pedicle length of 6 cm.
  - The average arterial diameter is 2 mm.
- The artery is accompanied by two venae comitantes, which may join or drain separately, with an average diameter of 1.5–2 mm.
- If skin is harvested with this flap, the blood supply is based on musculocutaneous perforators, with dominant perforators entering the muscle at the upper third.
- The vascular anatomy of the gracilis is consistent and, although it can reliably be harvested as a myocutaneous flap, there has been variability described in the size of its musculocutaneous perforators. Therefore, it more commonly is harvested as a muscle-only flap for use in facial reanimation or lip reconstruction procedures.

A. Badhey
Department of Otolaryngology- Head and Neck Surgery, UMass Chan Medical School, Worcester, MA, USA

A. L. Tang (✉)
Department of Otolaryngology- Head and Neck Surgery, University of Cincinnati Medical School, Cincinnati, OH, USA
e-mail: tangac@ucmail.uc.edu

R. Rezaee, A. Tamaki (eds.), *Local, Regional, and Free Flaps for Head and Neck Reconstruction*,
https://doi.org/10.1007/978-3-032-03211-9_19

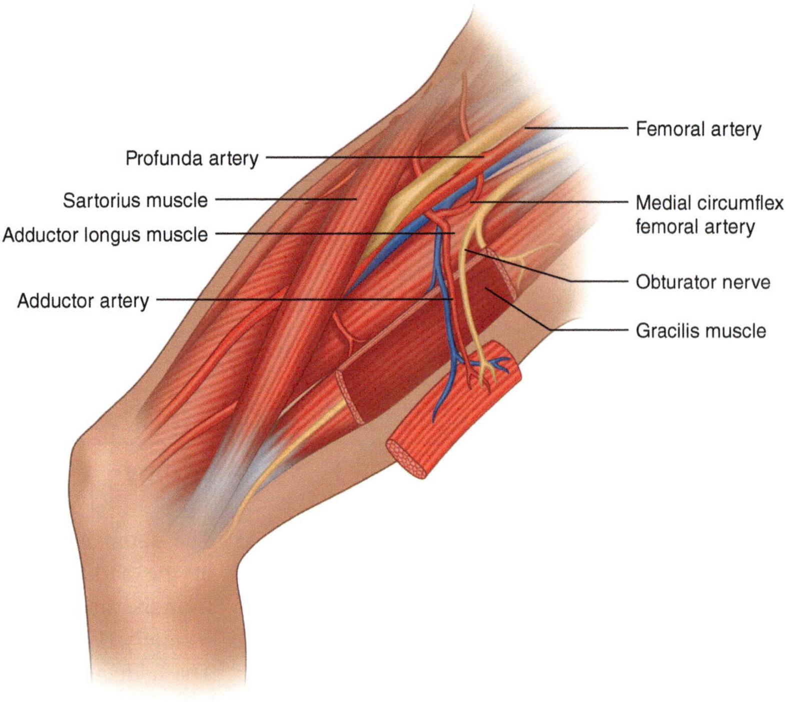

Fig. 19.1 The adductor artery runs along the adductor longus muscle before entering the gracilis muscle. Motor input to the gracilis flap is provided by the anterior branch of the obturator nerve, which enters the muscle superior to the entry point of the vascular pedicle

- Motor input to the gracilis muscle is provided by the anterior branch of the obturator nerve, which enters the muscle obliquely 2–3 cm superior to the entry point of the vascular pedicle. The nerve can also be traced between the adductor longus and brevis muscle to increase length [6].

Preoperative Care

- Assess for history of regional scars from prior surgery or trauma that may compromise vascular anatomy or perfusion to the skin.
- Consider hair-bearing portions prior to harvest if harvesting as a myocutaneous flap.

Special Instruments and Positioning

- Lithotomy or simple frog leg position with leg flexed and abducted.
- Expose from the pubic tubercle to the medial condyle.

Modifications

- Can be harvested with a skin paddle in conjunction with facial nerve reanimation (e.g., invasive skin cancer overlying the parotid region requiring facial nerve sacrifice).
- Can be harvested in different segments as a multi-paddle for multi-vector reanimation.
  - Muscle placed in different points along the zygoma will provide different smile excursions.
- Superiorly and inferior edges of the muscle can be transected with a gastrointestinal anastomosis stapler or suture oversewn to create a neotendon [2–5, 7, 9].

Pitfalls and Complications

- Short pedicle length.
- Leg adduction weakness is possible, but morbidity is limited due to the remaining adductor muscles.
- Smaller pedicle caliber leading to more complex microsurgical technique.

- At times the pedicle can travel through the adductor longus, and a small segment of muscle dissection is required to permit adequate pedicle length and dissection to the profunda femoris system.

Postoperative Care

- Reapproximate fascia of the adductor longus and magnus muscle.
- Elevate operated leg.
- One closed suction drain with removal after 3–5 days based on output [8].
- Can take up to 12 months for swelling within the face to subside [9].

Tissue type: *Muscular, musculocutaneous*
Artery: *Gracilis branch of the adductor artery*
Vein: *Venae comitantes*
Nerve: *Obturator nerve*
Pedicle length: 6 cm
Flap size: *30 cm length × 4–5 cm in width*

Operative Procedure

1. Surgical prep from the pubis to below the knee with the leg in the flexed, abducted, and externally rotated position.
   * The adductor longus becomes taught in this position and can be palpated and skin landmarks seen.
2. Draw a line from the origin of the gracilis (posterior to the adductor longus muscle), from the pubic tubercle to the medial femoral condyle.
3. The skin incision is placed 2–3 cm posterior to this line in the proximal/superior aspect of the thigh. Incise through the skin and subcutaneous tissue down to the muscle.
4. The gracilis is the most superficial of the adductor muscles and is located between the adductor longus anteriorly and the adductor magnus muscle posteriorly (Fig. 19.1).
   * It is the only muscle of the adductors that crosses the knee.
   * The sartorius muscle is also a helpful landmark as it is located above the gracilis in the midthigh.
5. After the gracilis muscle belly is identified, the pedicle is found on the deep surface, approximately 8–10 cm from the pubic tubercle, between the adductor longus and magnus.
   * The pedicle may be dissected through the adductor longus muscle to maximize length.
6. If reinnervation is planned, the anterior branch of the obturator nerve can be found 2–3 cm proximal to the vascular pedicle.
7. Divide the muscle, either through the same incision or through a separate incision distally at the pes anserinus of the knee.
8. Close the donor harvest site primarily, including reapproximating the fascia of the adductor longus and magnus. A drain is placed prior to closure.

Disclosure Statement No conflicts of interest to disclose.

References

1. Harii K, Ohmori K, Torii S. Free gracilis muscle transplantation with micro-vascular anastomoses for the treatment of facial paralysis. A preliminary report. Plast Reconstr Surg. 1976;57:133–43.
2. Azizzadeh B, Pettijohn KJ. The gracilis free flap. Facial Plast Surg Clin North Am. 2016;24(1):47–60. https://doi.org/10.1016/j.fsc.2015.09.002. PMID: 26611701
3. Roy M, Corkum J, Shah P, Borschel GH, Ho ES, Zuker RM, et al. Effectiveness and safety of the use of gracilis muscle for dynamic smile restoration in facial paralysis: a systematic review and meta-analysis. J Plast Reconstr Aesthet Surg. 2019;72:1254–64.
4. Chiesa-Estomba CM, González-García JÁ, Piazza C, Mayo-Yanez M, Grammatica A, Lechien JR, Din TF, Karkos P, García-Iza L, Ayad T. Gracilis free flap in head and neck reconstruction beyond facial palsy reanimation. Acta Otorrinolaringol Esp (Engl Ed). 2022;73(5):310–22. https://doi.org/10.1016/j.otoeng.2022.01.003. PMID: 36113921
5. O'Brien BM, Pederson WC, Khazanchi R, et al. Results of management of facial palsy with microvascular free-muscle transfer. Plast Reconstr Surg. 1990;86(1):12–22.
6. Magden O, Tayfur V, Edizer M, et al. Anatomy of gracilis muscle flap. J Craniofac Surg. 2010;21(6):1948–50.

7. Bae YC, Zuker RM, Manktelow RT, et al. A comparison of commissure excursion following gracilis muscle transplantation for facial paralysis using a cross-face nerve graft versus the motor nerve to the masseter nerve. Plast Reconstr Surg. 2006;117(7):2407–13.
8. Lee LN, Susarla SM, Henstrom DK, et al. Surgical site infections after gracilis free flap reconstruction for facial paralysis. Otolaryngol Head Neck Surg. 2012;147(2):245–8.
9. Sassoon EM, Poole MD, Rushworth G. Reanimation for facial palsy using gracilis muscle grafts. Br J Plast Surg. 1991;44:195–200.

20 Iliac Crest Free Flap

Samuel J. Rubin and Mark L. Urken

History

- In 1979, Sanders and Mayou as well as Taylor et al. described the deep circumflex iliac artery (DCIA) and the deep circumflex iliac vein (DCIV) as the main blood supply for transfer of the ileum using free tissue microvascular reconstruction [1, 2].
- In 1984, Ramasastry et al. described the ascending branch of the deep circumflex iliac artery as a separate blood supply to the internal oblique muscle, allowing the transfer of two separate soft tissue flaps [3].
- Shenaq et al. described the use of the iliac crest–internal oblique free flap for reconstruction of complex craniofacial defects in 1988 [4].
- In 1989, Urken described the use of the iliac crest–internal oblique osteomyocutaneous flap for oromandibular reconstruction, and subsequently, implant supported dental rehabilitation [5–8].

S. J. Rubin
Division of Otolaryngology- Head and Neck Surgery, Allegheny Health Network, Pittsburgh, PA, USA

M. L. Urken (✉)
THANC (Thyroid, Head and Neck Cancer) Foundation, New York, NY, USA

Department of Otolaryngology- Head and Neck Surgery, Icahn School of Medicine at Mount Sinai, New York, NY, USA
e-mail: Urken@mountsinai.org

Indications and Benefits

- Reconstruction of both oral cavity composite defects as well as palatomaxillary defects, especially when reconstruction of vertical height such as orbital rim is required [9, 10].
- Can be used to reconstruct multiple mandibular defects including both hemi-mandible defects using a single segment [11], as well as anterior defects.
  - The anterior superior iliac spine (ASIS) can be used to reconstruct the angle of the neomandible.
  - Anterior defects can be reconstructed using multiple opening osteotomies.
- Potential to harvest a large volume of bone, greater than that of the fibula, scapula, or radius [12].
  - Maximum of 16 cm in bone length.
  - Two layers of cortical bone and cancellous bone, which makes this bone ideal for endosteal dental implants.
- Ideal for reconstruction of composite defects.
- Potential to harvest a large volume of soft tissue including the internal oblique muscle and skin.
- Due to the axial blood supply of the internal oblique muscle in 80% of cases, the muscle can be rotated in three dimensions in relation to the iliac crest.
- Consistent anatomy (except variability in

R. Rezaee, A. Tamaki (eds.), *Local, Regional, and Free Flaps for Head and Neck Reconstruction*,
https://doi.org/10.1007/978-3-032-03211-9_20

branching pattern of the ascending branch of the DCIA).

Anatomy

- The main vascular supply to the iliac crest is the DCIA, which is a branch of the external iliac artery and originates a few centimeters above the inguinal ligament (Fig. 20.1).
  - The DCIA courses from its takeoff from the external iliac artery to the anterior superior iliac spine (ASIS) and then runs in a

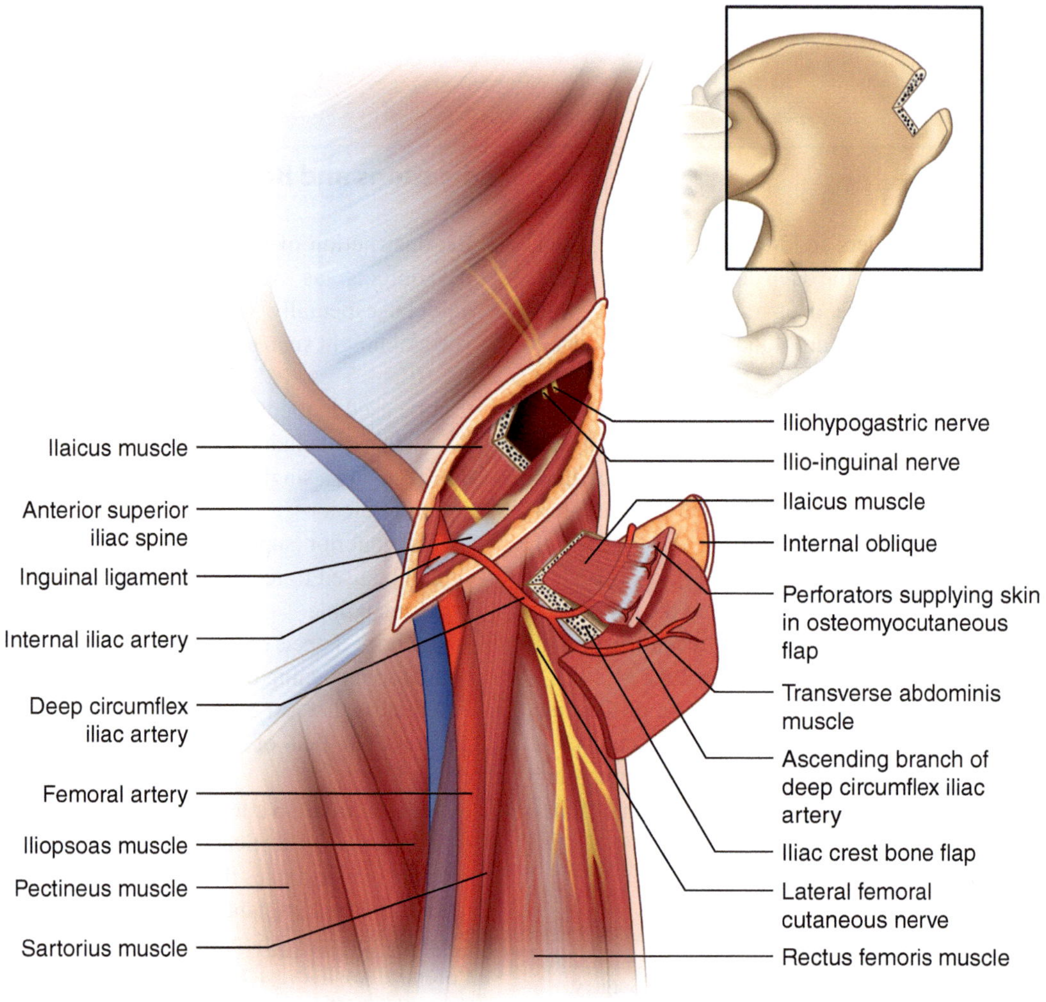

Fig. 20.1 Deep circumflex iliac artery (DCIA) originates a few centimeters above the inguinal ligament and supplies the iliac crest with both endosteal and periosteal vessels. The DCIA perforators traverses the external oblique, internal oblique, and transverse abdominis muscle before supplying the skin. The lateral femoral cutaneous nerve crosses medial to the anterior superior iliac spine, either superficial or deep to the DCIA pedicle

groove along the iliac crest superficial to the iliacus and deep to the transversus abdominis.
  - The DCIA supplies the iliac crest with both endosteal and periosteal vessels.
- Myocutaneous perforators from the DCIA traverse all three muscle layers (external oblique, internal oblique, transversus abdominus) (Fig. 20.1).
  - DCIA cutaneous perforators are located on the superior aspect of the iliac crest, 5–10.5 cm posterior to the ASIS [13].
- The DCIA gives off an ascending branch that travels through the transversus abdominus muscle and supplies the internal oblique muscle.
- There is variability in the branching patterning of the ascending branch of the DCIA [3, 14]:
  - 65% originate from the DCIA within 1 cm medial to the ASIS.
  - 15% originate 2–4 cm medial from the ASIS.
  - 20% of the internal oblique is supplied by multiple small branches and no dominant ascending branch.
- Deep circumflex iliac vein (DCIV) is usually composed of two venae comitantes that merge before entry into the external iliac vein.
  - The ascending branch of the DCIV runs in parallel with the artery and joins with the DCIV prior to entry into the external iliac vein.
- The flap is not sensate, but there are multiple nerves in the anatomical region that may be encountered during harvest.
  - Internal oblique muscle receives nerve supply from lower thoracic nerves, T8 to T12, iliohypogastric, and ilioinguinal nerves.
  - Lateral femoral cutaneous nerve exits the pelvic region and travels in a course medial to the ASIS.
  - Femoral nerve runs in a deep plane lateral to the external iliac artery and vein.

Preoperative Care

- Evaluate for history of abdominal surgeries, which may weaken abdominal wall or result in altered perfusion of the bone and skin paddle.
- In cases when the patient had a history of abdominal surgery or a hernia near the donor site, one should consider an alternative donor site.
- There is no preoperative imaging necessary for evaluation of DCIA/DCIV.

Special Instruments and Positioning

- Patient is positioned supine. The patient is prepped from midline of the abdomen to the midaxillary line and from the level of the 12th rib to the ipsilateral upper thigh.
- Large retractors such as Deaver retractors to retract abdominal fat and muscles.
- Synthetic mesh to support abdominal wall and decrease risk of hernia formation after harvest of internal oblique muscle.

Modifications

- Iliac crest osteocutaneous flap where a skin paddle is harvested with bone.
- Iliac crest osteomyocutaneous flap (iliac crest–internal oblique flap), including harvest of entire internal oblique muscle.
- Iliac crest myo-osseus flap, including partial harvest of the internal oblique muscle.
- Partial thickness osteocutaneous flap where the inner table of the iliac bone is harvested in the sagittal orientation.

Pitfalls and Complications

- Iliac crest osteomyocutaneous flap is not ideal when the cutaneous defect extends above the level of the lateral commissure when also reconstructing the mandible because of the negative effect on the vascular supply when stretching the skin paddle.
- The ascending branch of the DCIA may arise within 1–2 cm of the external iliac artery

approximately 5% of the time. In these situations, it may be necessary to treat the two vessels as separate pedicles.

- Possible duplication of the DCIA. A microvascular clamp should be placed on each artery to determine which pedicle is dominant prior to harvest of the composite flap.
- If the transversus abdominus muscle is thin, synthetic mesh may be needed to augment the closure of the abdominal wall and limit the risk of hernia formation.
- Attention must be paid to vital structures such as the femoral nerve and the intraperitoneal contents during harvest.
- Blood supply to the soft tissue may be compromised for a number of reasons:
  - Not incorporating enough perforators to the skin paddle.
  - Twisting of the skin paddle in relation to the iliac bone during inset causing poor perfusion.
  - Not preserving adequate cuff of the muscle layers of the abdominal wall, which may compromise the circulation to the skin.

Postoperative Care

- Progressive mobilization starting on postoperative day 3–4.
- Placement of pillows under the ipsilateral knee to the donor site to decrease tension on the abdominal wall closure.
- Patient is at risk of postoperative ileus, and therefore must be monitored for bowel sounds prior to starting nutrition.

Tissue type: *Myo-osseus, osseus (full thickness or split thickness), osteocutaneous, osteomyocutaneous*
Artery: *Deep circumflex iliac artery*
Vein: *Deep circumflex iliac vein*
Nerve: *Non-sensate flap (Can use lateral femoral cutaneous nerve as free nerve graft)*
Pedicle length: *5–7 cm*
Flap size: *16 cm of bone, entire internal oblique muscle; skin flap maximum size limited by ability for primary closure of abdomen (size not clearly defined)*

Operative Procedure

Iliac Crest Flap

1. The inguinal ligament and ASIS are palpated and marked.
2. If a skin paddle is going to be harvested, then an oval-shaped skin paddle should be designed along the axis of the iliac crest with the medial extent at the level of the ASIS.

   * The limitation in size of the skin paddle is based on the ability to close the abdomen primarily.
3. An incision is made through the cephalic portion of the skin paddle down to the level of the external oblique. Careful dissection should be performed in the plane between the subcutaneous tissue and the external oblique muscle to identify and preserve dominant myocutaneous perforators, which need to be maintained to preserve vascularity to the skin.
4. The external oblique and overlying fascia are incised leaving a cuff of muscle of approximately 2 cm attached to the inner table of the ilium.
5. An incision is made through the internal oblique muscle leaving 2 cm of muscle attached to the ilium. Cuts are made further away from the ilium in cases where the internal oblique muscle is to be harvested with the flap.
6. The ascending branch of the DCIA and DCIV are identified deep to the internal oblique and traced retrograde through the transversus abdominis muscle to the junction with the DCIA/DCIV and then, ultimately, the external iliac vessels.
7. The transversus abdominis is incised laterally leaving 2 cm attached to the inner table of the ilium, which exposes preperitoneal fat and the iliacus. This step will also expose the lateral femoral cutaneous nerve.

8. The iliacus is transected to expose the inner table of the ilium, leaving at least 2 cm of muscle attached to preserve the DCIA/DCIV.
9. Lateral dissection occurs by incising along the inferolateral border of the skin paddle to the level of the tensor fascia lata and the gluteus medius.
10. Dissection is performed along the lateral aspect of the iliac bone starting at the posterolateral lip of the iliac crest to provide exposure of the outer table of the ilium. This portion of the dissection is carried out to the required depth to harvest the required amount of bone.
11. The DCIA/DCIV are dissected between the ASIS and takeoff from the external iliac vessels. The DCIA enters the external iliac artery directly, while the DCIV takes a more cephalad course before entering the external iliac vein.
12. The iliopsoas and sartorius muscles are transected.
13. Using deep retractors to protect the abdominal content, osteotomies are performed from the lateral exposure.

    * Care must be taken to protect to the DCIA/DCIV when making the medial bone cuts.
14. Once the flap is isolated on the DCIA/DCIV pedicle, all components of the flap should be assessed for adequacy of the circulation.
15. The DCIA/DCIV are then ligated to complete the harvest.
16. Copious irrigation and hemostasis is performed.
17. Synthetic mesh is often used to augment the abdominal wall closure when there is concern for weakening of the abdominal wall, especially when the internal oblique muscle is harvested in addition to the iliac crest. *(See below for section on closure of abdominal wall with synthetic mesh.)*
18. If the internal oblique muscle is preserved, the transversus abdominis and internal oblique muscle are sutured to the iliacus muscle.

    * Drill holes may be performed through the cut margin of the iliac bone through which sutures are placed which traverse the iliacus, transversus abdominis, and internal oblique muscles to strengthen the closure.
19. The external oblique muscle and aponeurosis are sutured to the tensor fascia lata and tendon of the gluteus medius.
20. Layered approximation of the subcutaneous tissue and skin is performed.

Iliac Crest–Internal Oblique Flap

1. A skin paddle is designed along an axis drawn from the ASIS to the inferior border of the scapula.
2. The cephalic portion of the skin paddle is incised down to the level of the external oblique muscle.
3. Careful dissection should be performed in the plane between the subcutaneous tissue and the external oblique muscle to identify and preserve dominant myocutaneous perforators, which need to be maintained to preserve vascularity to the skin (Fig. 20.1).
4. The external oblique is incised 2.5–3 cm above the iliac crest.

    * The external oblique muscle should not be dissected in the caudal direction off of the internal oblique. This may compromise the perforators that pass through the muscle layers.
5. The perimeter of the internal oblique is incised and raised off the transversus abdominis in a cephalad to caudal direction while maintaining the inferior attachments to the iliac crest.
6. The ascending branch of the DCIA/DCIV is identified on the deep aspect of the internal oblique muscle and traced to its junction with the external iliac vessels. *(See above in Iliac Crest Flap section for remainder of surgical steps for harvest.)*

Synthetic Mesh Closure of Abdominal Wall

Synthetic mesh is placed in between the transversus abdominis muscle and external oblique and attached to the iliac crest below and internal oblique on the remaining sides.

1. Drill holes are made in the iliac bone and permanent sutures are passed through the drill holes → iliacus → transversus abdominis → synthetic mesh.
   * All sutures are placed while protecting the peritoneal contents with ribbon retractors.
   * All sutures are placed and then tied.
2. The mesh is then sutured to the medial, superior, and posterior margins of the internal oblique muscle and aponeurosis.

Disclosure Statement Mark Urken is the Medical Director of the THANC foundation.

References

1. Taylor GI, Townsend P, Corlett R. Superiority of the deep circumflex iliac vessels as the supply for free groin flaps. Clinical work. Plast Reconstr Surg. 1979;64(6):745–59.
2. Sanders R, Mayou BJ. A new vascularized bone graft transferred by microvascular anastomosis as a free flap. Br J Surg. 1979;66(11):787–8.
3. Ramasastry SS, Granick MS, Futrell JW. Clinical anatomy of the internal oblique muscle. J Reconstr Microsurg. 1986;2(2):117–22.
4. Shenaq SM. Reconstruction of complex cranial and craniofacial defects utilizing iliac crest-internal oblique microsurgical free flap. Microsurgery. 1988;9(2):154–8.
5. Urken ML, Vickery C, Weinberg H, Buchbinder D, Biller HF. The internal oblique-iliac crest osseomyocutaneous microvascular free flap in head and neck reconstruction. J Reconstr Microsurg. 1989;5(3):203–14. discussion 215-216
6. Urken ML, Vickery C, Weinberg H, Buchbinder D, Lawson W, Biller HF. The internal oblique-iliac crest osseomyocutaneous free flap in oromandibular reconstruction. Report of 20 cases. Arch Otolaryngol Head Neck Surg. 1989;115(3):339–49.
7. Urken ML, Weinberg H, Vickery C, Buchbinder D, Lawson W, Biller HF. The internal oblique-iliac crest free flap in composite defects of the oral cavity involving bone, skin, and mucosa. Laryngoscope. 1991;101(3):257–70.
8. Moscoso JF, Urken ML. The iliac crest composite flap for oromandibular reconstruction. Otolaryngol Clin N Am. 1994;27(6):1097–117.
9. Urken ML, Roche AM, Kiplagat KJ, et al. Comprehensive approach to functional palatomaxillary reconstruction using regional and free tissue transfer: report of reconstructive and prosthodontic outcomes of 140 patients. Head Neck. 2018;40(8):1639–66.
10. Genden EM, Wallace D, Buchbinder D, Okay D, Urken ML. Iliac crest internal oblique osteomusculocutaneous free flap reconstruction of the postablative palatomaxillary defect. Arch Otolaryngol Head Neck Surg. 2001;127(7):854–61.
11. Manchester WM. Immediate reconstruction of the mandible and temporomandibular joint. Br J Plast Surg. 1965;18:291–303.
12. Moscoso JF, Keller J, Genden E, et al. Vascularized bone flaps in oromandibular reconstruction. A comparative anatomic study of bone stock from various donor sites to assess suitability for enosseous dental implants. Arch Otolaryngol Head Neck Surg. 1994;120(1):36–43.
13. Bergeron L, Tang M, Morris SF. The anatomical basis of the deep circumflex iliac artery perforator flap with iliac crest. Plast Reconstr Surg. 2007;120(1):252–8.
14. Taylor GI, Townsend P, Corlett R. Superiority of the deep circumflex iliac vessels as the supply for free groin flaps. Plast Reconstr Surg. 1979;64(5):595–604.

21 Jejunal Free Flap

Melina Windon, Linda X. Yin, and Steven B. Chinn

History

- César Roux, an accomplished Swiss surgeon, described the first human use of a pedicled jejunum flap for esophageal reconstruction in 1907 [1].
- In the 1930s–1940s, many surgeons [2, 3] reported using the Roux pedicled jejunal method, noting variability in small bowel vascular anatomy and high rates of flap loss.
- Free vascularized transfer of small bowel, first reported by Carrel in 1907 [4], was adopted by Longmire [5] in 1947 for the Roux jejunal flap. This allowed for vascular augmentation of the jejunal flap through microvascular anastomosis of the jejunal mesenteric vessels to donor vessels in the neck or chest, thus creating the "supercharged" jejunal flap.
- In the 1950s–1960s, the use of the jejunal free flap was popularized, establishing it as a useful reconstructive tool after total laryngopharyngectomy [6].

Indications and Benefits

- Primary indication is for circumferential pharyngoesophageal reconstruction and restoration of the upper aerodigestive tract.
  - Defects may be the result of hypopharyngeal, laryngeal, or upper esophageal malignancies, congenital anomalies including esophageal atresia or tracheoesophageal fistula, or severe pharyngoesophageal stenosis that has failed more conservative measures.
  - Jejunal free flap may also be used for oral cavity and oropharyngeal reconstruction as a patch or tube, although this is less common in the modern era due to the popularity of other fasciocutaneous free flaps.
- The jejunum is ideal for pharyngoesophageal reconstruction because it is a lubricated, tubular structure lined with mucosa and it has intrinsic peristaltic activity similar to the native esophagus [7].
  - Advantages of the jejunal free flap include rapid healing, as well as lack of functional

M. Windon
Department of Otolaryngology- Head and Neck Surgery, University of Kentucky, Lexington, KY, USA

L. X. Yin
Mayo Clinic Rochester, Rochester, MN, USA

S. B. Chinn (✉)
Department of Otolaryngology- Head and Neck Surgery, University of Michigan, Ann Arbor, MI, USA

Rogel Cancer Center, University of Michigan, Ann Arbor, MI, USA
e-mail: schinn@umich.edu

R. Rezaee, A. Tamaki (eds.), *Local, Regional, and Free Flaps for Head and Neck Reconstruction*, https://doi.org/10.1007/978-3-032-03211-9_21

sequelae to the donor site.
- Rate of anastomotic stricture may be less compared to fasciocutaneous free flaps [8].
- Jejunum avoids issues with gastric pull-up including reflux, early satiety, and reach [9].

Anatomy

- The jejunum is the second part of the small bowel. It is 4 cm in diameter [11] and starts at the Ligament of Treitz [12] distal to the duodenum and runs for about 250 cm. It is suspended to the abdominal wall by the mesentery [6], which is 15 cm wide [11].
- Layers of the jejunum from the outside in are the serosa, muscle (outer longitudinal and inner circular muscle layers), the myenteric neural plexus (Auerbach's and Meissner's), submucosa, glands, and mucosa [6].
- Vascular blood supply to the jejunum is via branches of the superior mesenteric artery (SMA). Each jejunal artery branch supplies a segment of the jejunum up to 25 cm in length. Each artery splits into two marginal vessels and unites with adjacent branches to form vascular arcades within the mesentery and the mesenteric border of the bowel wall (Fig. 21.1) [6].
  - The arcades terminate in the vasa recta, capillaries that traverse the bowel wall between the muscle and mucosa, forming a submucosal plexus.
  - There are usually four to five branches from the SMA that supply the jejunum in the first 60 cm; however, this ranges from 1 to 5 [12, 13].
- Extrinsic innervation to the jejunum is via preganglionic parasympathetic and postganglionic sympathetic branches from the celiac plexus [6]. The nerves accompany the vessels in the mesentery entering the jejunum. Jejunal free flaps are typically not innervated due to the intrinsic innervation of the jejunum.
- Intrinsic innervation to the jejunum is via the myenteric plexus of Auerbach and the submucosal plexus of Meissner. Reflex arcs with afferents from the mucosa and efferents from

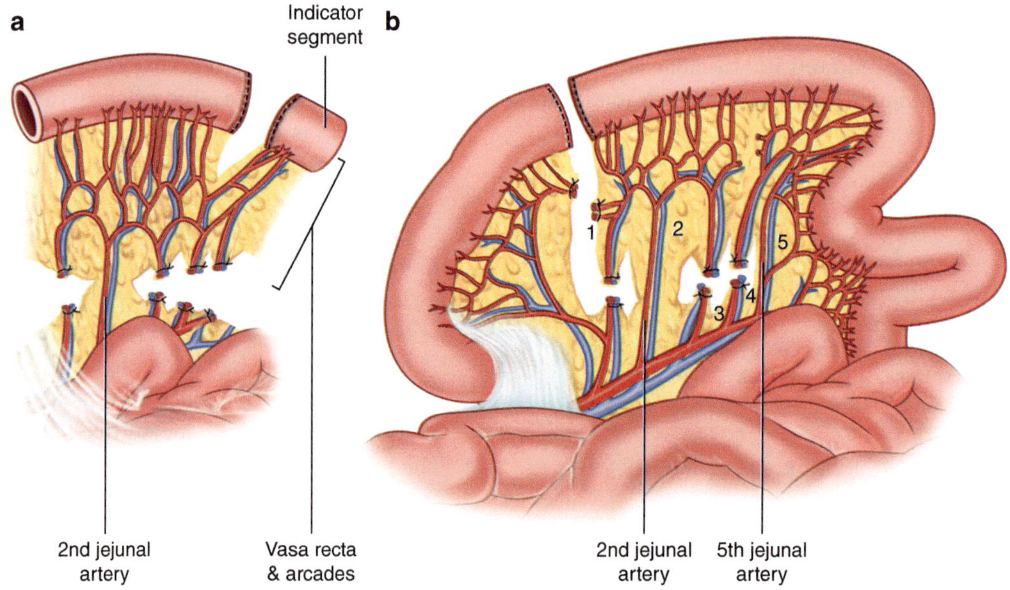

Fig. 21.1 Vascular blood supply to the jejunum is via branches of the superior mesenteric artery. Each jejunal artery branch supplies a segment of the jejunum up to 25 cm in length. (**a**) Free jejunum flap based on the second jejunal artery. A monitoring (indicator) segment may be exteriorized. (**b**) In a supercharged jejunum flap, the second jejunal artery is divided and re-anastomosed in the neck. The third and fourth jejunal arteries are ligated and the surrounding mesentery directed free from the bowel for length. The fifth jejunal artery is preserved as the pedicled portion of the flap

the motor fibers of the myenteric plexus allow for autonomous movements of the jejunum despite lack of extrinsic nerve supply [6].

Preoperative Care

- A multidisciplinary surgical team is key, since jejunal harvest is performed by a thoracic or general surgeon.
- Nutritional status optimization is crucial before surgery, as malnutrition is a significant risk factor for pharyngocutaneous fistula and anastomotic leak [14].
- No bowel prep is necessary before surgery [12, 15].
- In patients who are poor candidates for immediate pharyngoesophageal reconstruction, a pharyngostomal spit fistula can be created in the upper neck, and the cervical esophagus can be closed in a blind sac.
  - The patient is then fed through a feeding tube until medically optimized for reconstruction.
- Careful history should be obtained from the patient regarding any previous abdominal surgeries, laparoscopic or open. The position of previous percutaneous enteric feeding tubes should be identified and noted.
- Recipient vessel availability must be assessed prior to surgery. Updated cross-sectional neck imaging and a thorough surgical history should be obtained. Many patients requiring total pharyngoesophageal reconstruction have vessel depleted necks and/or a previous history of radiation.

Special Instruments and Positioning

- Salivary bypass tube may be used for stenting and diversion of saliva.
- Gastrointestinal anastomosis (GIA) stapler is helpful for jejunal harvest and a mechanical stapler is used by some at the distal anastomosis in the neck as well [16].
- Nasogastric tube should be placed for decompression, and a jejunostomy tube should be placed for enteric feeding.
- Patient positioned supine, with both arms tucked, and prepped widely from the neck down to the chest and abdomen.

Modifications

- Can be harvested as a free flap. A maximum of 25 cm of jejunum based off a single arcade branch of artery and vein can be harvested. Laparoscopic harvest technique can be considered.
- Can be harvested as a pedicled "supercharged" flap. This is most helpful for long segment esophageal or pharyngoesophageal reconstruction, particularly in salvage cases when a gastric conduit cannot be used or cannot provide enough length [12].
  - In this technique, the jejunum is divided after the segment supplied by the first branch off the SMA.
  - Typically, the second jejunal branch off the SMA is used for microvascular anastomosis in the neck or chest.
  - The third or even the fourth branches can be taken down as backup vessels for microvascular anastomosis, and to achieve increased mobility on the jejunum. The most distal branch(es) are preserved on the primary blood supply from the SMA.
  - The conduit can be pulled up to the neck or chest through an intrathoracic route [13].
  - With this technique, the entire cervical and thoracic esophagus can be replaced [9]. The reach has been described to the skull base [17].

Pitfalls and Complications

- Disadvantages include the requirement of a general or thoracic surgery team and added morbidity and prolonged recovery associated with open abdominal surgery [10].
- Shorter vascular pedicle and shorter tolerance for ischemia time compared to other available flaps.
- Risk of anastomotic leak in the neck or the abdomen.

- Postoperative regurgitation and dysphagia.
- Intra-abdominal bleeding and hematoma from the mesentery.
- Postoperative ileus.
  - This should be aggressively managed as vomiting or retching poses a threat to the fresh jejunopharyngeal and/or jejunoesophageal anastomoses.
- Compared to tubed fasciocutaneous free flaps used in pharyngoesophageal reconstruction, tracheoesophageal speech following jejunal flaps has been described as having a "wet" sound.
  - Tubed skin flaps may have better speech and swallowing function [18].
- Unexpected ligation of the jejunal vessels beyond the main vessel bifurcation is possible, especially in obese patients.
  - If this occurs, proceed with anastomosis with the intact branch even though it is beyond the bifurcation, as the majority of the bowel segment can be viable on a single branch of artery. Assess the flap after revascularization, and trim any part of the bowel that does not appear viable [6].

Postoperative Care

- Nasogastric tube placed at the time of surgery should be kept on low suction to decompress the stomach and minimize the risk of reflux into the fresh anastomosis site.
  - Once bowel function has returned to normal and output is diminished through the gastric tube, it can be clamped and eventually removed.
- After confirmation of bowel sounds, the patient can be fed enterically through the jejunostomy tube.
- The monitoring segment of bowel (indicator flap) can be ligated at 1 week after surgery if the flap has shown signs of healthy perfusion.
- Arterial thrombus must be managed urgently as the bowel is particularly sensitive to ischemia [19, 20].
- A swallow study can be obtained 2 weeks after surgery to assess for small anastomotic leaks prior to starting and oral diet at the discretion of the reconstructive surgeon.
- Anastomotic leaks, most of which occur at the proximal anastomosis, resolve with conservative management. Distal anastomotic leaks are more likely to require reoperation [21].

Tissue type: *Visceral (intestinal mucosa, muscle, and serosa, as well as mesenteric fat)*
Artery: *Jejunal arteries arising from the superior mesenteric artery*
Vein: *Jejunal veins*
Nerve: *None (intrinsic innervation)*
Pedicle length: *7–11 cm*[6]
Flap size: *In free flap transfer, up to a 25-cm-long segment of jejunum can be harvested off a single jejunal artery and vein; in a "supercharged" jejunal flap, the length of reach of the jejunum is limited by the number of arcades left pedicled on the superior mesenteric artery*

Operative Procedure

Jejunal Free Flap

1. The jejunum is accessed through a vertical upper midline abdominal incision.
2. The duodenal jejunal flexure is located, and the jejunal branches of the SMA inspected via transillumination. The second jejunal branch is most commonly selected for microvascular anastomosis given its length, though the third or fourth may be suitable as well (Fig. 21.1b) [11].
3. The desired length of intestine centered on the selected pedicle is marked, and the intestine divided with a stapler. The proximal portion of the flap is marked clearly with a suture to maintain isoperistaltic orientation at inset.
4. The adjacent arcades are ligated, and the mesentery is divided, maximizing preservation of the vasa recta.
5. The selected jejunal artery is carefully dissected up to its origin at the SMA [11].

6. The jejunum should be carefully inspected for signs of perfusion, including pink color, peristalsis, and Doppler signal on the vasa recta.
7. The pedicle is divided and the jejunum bathed in cold normal saline.
8. The jejunal continuity is reestablished end-to-end, and a jejunostomy tube placed for feeding [11].
9. The abdomen in closed in the standard fashion, over closed suction drains.
10. Taking care to minimize ischemia time, the flap is transferred to the recipient bed and oriented in the isoperistaltic orientation. The microvascular anastomosis is performed [22]. The proximal pharyngojejunal anastomosis may be performed prior to the microvascular anastomosis.
11. The staple line is trimmed off of the jejunum and the antimesenteric side of the bowel incised to flute the bowel for closure. The proximal anastomosis is performed in 1 or 2 layers with sutures thrown 5 mm apart. A double-layered closure may lower the fistula rate. The distal anastomosis is performed in a single layer to prevent stricture [21].

    * If the distal anastomosis is low, a stapler can be employed [9].

    * The flap inset may be performed with the head in neutral position to minimize redundancy in the alimentary tract.
12. A segment of distal jejunum is divided and left pedicled onto the blood supply and brought out of the lateral neck as a reporter segment to monitor for flap perfusion based on color, peristalsis, and Doppler signal (indicator flap) (Fig. 21.1a). After 5–7 days, the vascular pedicle to this segment can be carefully clipped or tied, and the skin overclosed [11].

Supercharged Jejunal Interposition

1. Same as Steps 1–4 above.
2. The second jejunal artery is skeletonized to the SMA origin.
3. The retrosternal (for delayed reconstruction) or retrocardiac space (for immediate reconstruction) is dissected to allow for tunneling.

    * Additional measures to avoid kinking in the retrosternal route must be taken. These include resection of the manubrium, clavicular head, and first rib. This allows access to the internal mammary vessels.
4. Division of the distal jejunum for additional mobility of the pedicled segment is an option during immediate reconstruction. The small bowel is then closed with a jejunojejunostomy.
5. An Acland clamp is placed on the second jejunal artery, and the pedicle is divided.
6. The third and fourth jejunal arteries are ligated and the surrounding mesentery dissected free from the bowel for length.
7. The fifth jejunal artery is carefully preserved as the pedicled portion of the flap.
8. The jejunum is divided and laid across the chest up to the neck to assess for reach. The mesentery can be divided up to the bowel between the third and fourth jejunal arteries in order to unfurl its length.
9. The flap is placed into a bag and carefully passed through the chest, taking care not to kink or denude the serosa.
10. Microvascular anastomosis is performed to reestablish vascular flow to the watershed area in the proximal jejunum.
11. The distal jejunal flap, if the distal jejunum was divided, is either anastomosed to the gastric remnant or to the proximal jejunum as a Roux limb. If only the proximal jejunum was divided, the proximal small bowel is anastomosed end-to-side into the jejunum at a more distal location.
12. A proximal monitoring segment (indicator flap) may be exteriorized [17].
13. The abdomen is closed in the standard fashion, over closed suction drains.

Disclosure Statement No conflicts of interest to disclose.

References

1. Roux C. A new operation for intractable obstruction of the esophagus (L'oesophago-jejuno-gastrosiose, nouvelle operation pour retrecissement infrachissable del'oesophagus). Semin Med. 1907;27:34–40.
2. Yudin SS. The surgical construction of 80 cases of artificial esophagus. Surg Gynecol Obstet. 1944;78:561–83.
3. Ochsner A, Owens N. Antethoracic oesophagoplasty for impermeable stricture of the oesophagus. Ann Surg. 1934;100(6):1055–91.
4. Carrel A. Surgery of blood vessels, etc. Bull Hopkins Hosp. 1907;18:18.
5. Longmire WP Jr. A modification of the Roux technique for antethoracic esophageal reconstruction. Surgery. 1947;22(1):94–100.
6. Haughey BH. The jejunal free flap in oral cavity and pharyngeal reconstruction. Otolaryngol Clin N Am. 1994;27(6):1159–70.
7. Razdan SN, Albornoz CR, Matros E, Paty PB, Cordeiro PG. Free Jejunal flap for Pharyngoesophageal reconstruction in head and neck cancer patients: an evaluation of donor-site complications. J Reconstr Microsurg. 2015;31(9):643–6.
8. Wang S, Yang X, Peng X, Tang Q, Guo L, Tang X. Efficacy of free anterolateral thigh flap and free jejunum in reconstruction for hypopharyngeal and cervical esophagus. Zhong Nan Da Xue Xue Bao Yi Xue Ban. 2022;47(7):888–94.
9. Urken ML, Cheney ML, Blackwell KE, Harris JR, Hadlock TA, Futran N. Atlas of regional and free flaps for head and neck reconstruction: flap harvest and insetting. Wolters Kluwer Health; 2012.
10. Deschler DG, Herr MW, Kmiecik JR, Sethi R, Bunting G. Tracheoesophageal voice after total laryngopharyngectomy reconstruction: jejunum versus radial forearm free flap. Laryngoscope. 2015;125(12):2715–21.
11. Strauch B, Yu HL. Atlas of microvascular surgery: anatomy and operative techniques. Thieme; 2011.
12. Mohan AT, Mardini S, Blackmon SH. Supercharged Jejunal interposition. Thorac Surg Clin. 2022;32(4):529–40.
13. Yasuda T, Shiozaki H. Esophageal reconstruction using a pedicled jejunum with microvascular augmentation. Ann Thorac Cardiovasc Surg. 2011;17(2):103–9.
14. Mattioli F, Bettini M, Molteni G, et al. Analysis of risk factors for pharyngocutaneous fistula after total laryngectomy with particular focus on nutritional status. Acta Otorhinolaryngol Ital. 2015;35(4):243–8.
15. Benazzo M, Occhini A, Rossi V, Aresi G, Alessiani M. Jejunum free flap in hypopharynx reconstruction: case series. BMC Cancer. 2002;2(1):13.
16. Park J, Kang N, Oh SH, Lee SI, Song SH. The use of a mechanical stapler in Jejunal free flaps in Laryngopharyngectomy defects. Arch Plast Surg. 2015;42(6):815–8.
17. Mays AC, Yu P, Hofstetter W, et al. The supercharged Pedicled Jejunal flap for Total esophageal reconstruction: a retrospective review of 100 cases. Plast Reconstr Surg. 2019;144(5):1171–80.
18. Yu P, Lewin JS, Reece GP, Robb GL. Comparison of clinical and functional outcomes and hospital costs following pharyngoesophageal reconstruction with the anterolateral thigh free flap versus the jejunal flap. Plast Reconstr Surg. 2006;117(3):968–74.
19. Walker RJ, Parmar S, Praveen P, et al. Jejunal free flap for reconstruction of pharyngeal defects in patients with head and neck cancer-the Birmingham experience. Br J Oral Maxillofac Surg. 2014;52(2):106–10.
20. Reece GP, Bengtson BP, Schusterman MA. Reconstruction of the pharynx and cervical esophagus using free jejunal transfer. Clin Plast Surg. 1994;21(1):125–36.
21. Chang DW, Hussussian C, Lewin JS, Youssef AA, Robb GL, Reece GP. Analysis of pharyngocutaneous fistula following free jejunal transfer for total laryngopharyngectomy. Plast Reconstr Surg. 2002;109(5):1522–7.
22. Dash NR, Agarwal L, Singh CA, Thakar A. Use of free jejunal flap as a salvage procedure in the management of high corrosive esophageal re-strictures: an institutional experience and review of literature. Langenbeck's Arch Surg. 2022;407(7):2725–32.

Lateral Arm Free Flap

22

Janice L. Farlow and Stephen Y. Kang

History

- Song et al. first introduced the lateral arm fasciocutaneous flap in 1982 [1].

Indications and Benefits

- Versatile flap for a variety of soft tissue defects of the head and neck including the oral cavity, oropharynx, larynx, pharynx, and cutaneous defects.
- Good color match to facial skin and often non-hair-bearing.
- Thinner skin can be harvested from the distal upper arm, or thicker tissue from the proximal upper arm can be used depending on the reconstructive need.
- Compartmentalized adipose tissue allows for highly customized volume reconstruction that resists gravitational forces postoperatively [2].
- Provides access to two nerves for a neurotized flap and/or for nerve grafting.
- Reliable primary closure of donor site if width is limited to 6–8 cm or one-third of the arm's circumference.
  - Large flaps up to 11 × 18 cm have been described [3].
- Consistent anatomic landmarks for harvest.

Anatomy

- The lateral arm skin is supplied by 4–5 septocutaneous perforators arising from the posterior radial collateral artery, one of two terminal branches of the profunda brachii artery, which in turn arises from the brachial artery (Fig. 22.1).
  - Duplication of the profunda brachii has been reported in 4–12% of patients [4].
- The axis of the pedicle and the lateral intermuscular septum lie 1 cm posterior to the plane connecting the acromioclavicular joint or the deltoid insertion to the lateral epicondyle of the humerus. Of the landmarks, the deltoid insertion is often more readily and reliably palpable depending on the body habitus of the patient.
- The pedicle can be found in close approximation to the radial nerve between the triceps posteriorly and the brachialis and brachioradialis anteriorly.

J. L. Farlow
Department of Otolaryngology- Head and Neck Surgery, Indiana University School of Medicine, Indianapolis, IN, USA

S. Y. Kang (✉)
Department of Otolaryngology- Head and Neck Surgery, The James Cancer Hospital and Solove Research Institute, The Ohio State University, Columbus, OH, USA
e-mail: stephen.kang@osumc.edu

R. Rezaee, A. Tamaki (eds.), *Local, Regional, and Free Flaps for Head and Neck Reconstruction*,
https://doi.org/10.1007/978-3-032-03211-9_22

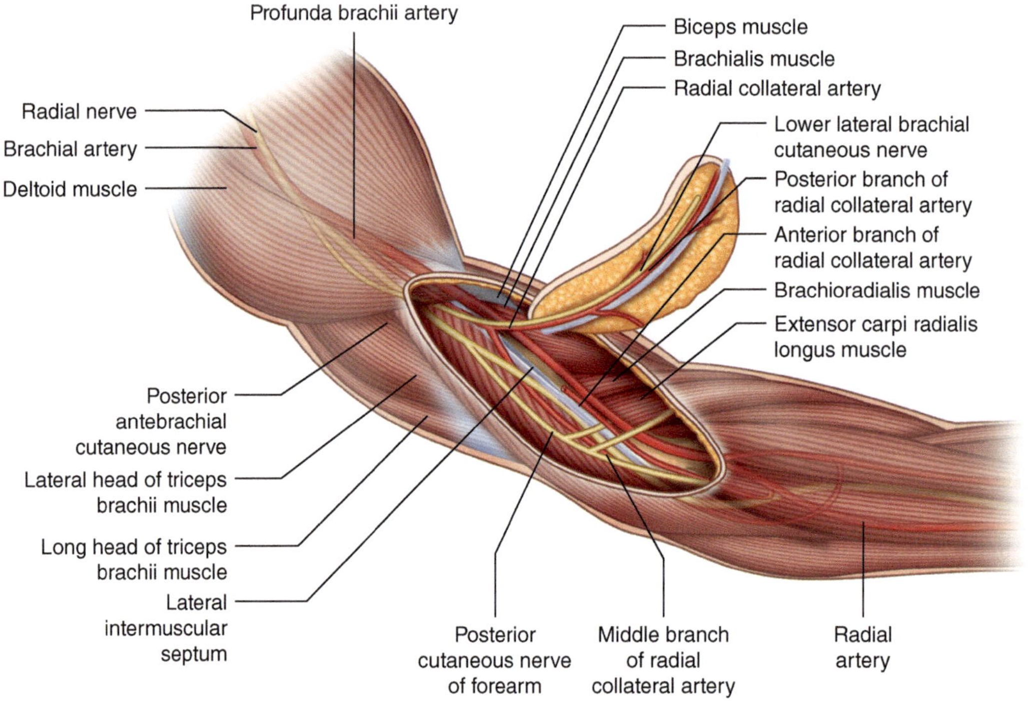

Fig. 22.1 The fasciocutaneous lateral arm flap is depicted, along with its arterial supply from the posterior radial collateral artery and its relationship with the intermuscular septum found just between the lateral head of the triceps brachii posteriorly and the brachialis/brachioradialis anteriorly. Two nerves emanating from the radial nerve available for harvest with the flap include the lower lateral brachial cutaneous nerve, or the posterior cutaneous nerve of the forearm

  - The average pedicle length is 7–8 cm, although an additional 6–8 cm can be obtained through an extended dissection under the triceps muscle [5].
  - At the level of the deltoid insertion, the posterior radial collateral artery has a diameter of 1.25–1.75 mm and widens to 1.75–2.7 mm just below its origin from the brachial artery [3].
- Two nerves arising from the radial nerve can be found when harvesting the lateral arm flap.
  - The posterior cutaneous nerve of the arm supplies sensation to the flap and can be used to create a neurotized flap.
  - The posterior cutaneous nerve to the forearm supplies sensation to the lateral forearm and is found in the fascia anterior to the lateral epicondyle of the humerus. This can be harvested along with any of its several branches for nerve grafting.
- Venous drainage consists of a deep system of two venae comitantes, which are approximately 2.5 mm in diameter [6], as well as a superficial system draining to the cephalic vein. In the authors' experience, generally only the deep system is harvested and one vena is chosen for anastomosis if they do not converge into a common vena [2].

Preoperative Care

- A thorough history and examination for scars should be performed of the axilla and shoulder girdle to determine if prior surgery or trauma may compromise the flap.

Special Instruments and Positioning

- The arm is internally rotated, the elbow positioned on a stack of sterile towels, and the palm of the hand supported on the patient's abdomen to provide optimal access for harvest.
- Circumferential sterile prep of the hand and arm up to and including the shoulder and axilla is ideal. A stockinette can be used for padding and positioning of the hand and forearm.

Modifications

- For an extended cutaneous paddle, the proximal forearm skin up to 10–12 cm distal to the lateral condyle can be harvested based on the vascular plexus of the posterior elbow that is fed by the posterior radial collateral artery [7].
- If a wide cutaneous paddle is required, a long but thinner skin paddle can be harvested with the two skin islands juxtaposed to one another at inset [8].
- A segment of humerus up to 1 × 10 cm can be harvested with the lateral arm fasciocutaneous flap by preserving a cuff of triceps and brachioradialis on the lateral intermuscular septum [9]. The harvested width is limited to 1 cm to avoid humeral fracture.
- The triceps tendon can also be harvested with the lateral arm flap, as reported for extremity reconstruction [8].

Pitfalls and Complications

- Pedicle length is generally limited to 7–8 cm, and the pedicle consists of a smaller caliber artery and vein than other fasciocutaneous flaps, limiting recipient vessel options.
  - This mismatch can be mitigated by clear communication with the ablative team to preserve the facial or superior thyroid artery and vein in situ, if oncologically sound, as these vessels at their more distal extent or the superior laryngeal branches often have a similar caliber for anastomosis.
- Radial nerve palsies due to compressive dressings or tight closure have been reported [6].
- Theoretically, forearm extension may be limited due to partial disconnection of the triceps from the distal humerus [10].

Postoperative Care

- Limitation of heavy lifting and routine incision care is all that is necessary for fasciocutaneous harvests with primary closure of the donor site.
- One closed suction drain is placed with removal after 3–5 days based on output.

Tissue type: *Adipofascial, fasciocutaneous*
Artery: *Posterior radial collateral artery*
Vein: *Venae comitantes*
Nerve: *Posterior cutaneous nerve to the forearm, posterior cutaneous nerve of the arm*
Pedicle length: *7–8 cm unless dissection carried under the triceps muscle*
Flap size: *Up to 11 × 18 cm, although a width of 6–8 cm recommended for primary closure of donor site*

Operative Procedure

1. Mark a line connecting the acromioclavicular joint or the deltoid insertion to the lateral epicondyle of the humerus. The axis of the pedicle 1 cm posterior to this line is marked, and a Doppler can be used to identify septocutaneous perforators along the axis of the flap.
2. The cutaneous paddle is generally drawn centered over the distal humerus, allowing the harvest of thinner skin and a longer pedicle. A pinch test is used to determine the maximal width of the flap to allow primary closure of the defect, which is approximately one-third the circumference of the arm.

   * Extended cutaneous paddles have been reported, up to 10 cm proximal to the deltoid insertion and 10 cm distal to the lateral epicondyle [6].

3. Position the arm internally rotated with the palm of the hand resting on the abdomen. A tourniquet can be used for flap harvest but may interfere with proximal dissection of the pedicle.
4. Make the posterior incision through the skin, subcutaneous tissues, and down to the triceps fascia.

   * Undermining posteriorly to harvest a 1 cm cuff of adipose can provide tissue that ultimately lies under the line of inset, thus preventing a trapdoor deformity [2]. The same maneuver can be performed for the anterior incision.
5. Perform subfascial dissection to the lateral border of the lateral triceps head. At this point, septocutaneous perforators and their takeoff from the posterior radial collateral artery can be identified. Perforators to the triceps muscle itself should be sequentially ligated (Fig. 22.1).
6. Next, make the anterior incision through skin and subcutaneous tissue down to the fascia of the brachialis and brachioradialis.
7. Identify the posterior cutaneous nerve of the forearm (PCNF) in the distal fascia anterior to the lateral epicondyle. This can be followed for the desired length and branching pattern before dividing it distally. The distal incision can be extended to facilitate this dissection. The nerve can be kept attached to the flap for a vascularized nerve graft or, alternatively, separated for free cable grafting.

   * A nerve stimulator can be used to confirm that nerve branches are all sensory.
8. Palpate the distal humerus and divide the distal attachments of the lateral intermuscular septum from the bone sharply. The distal pedicle can then be ligated. Continue dissection of the pedicle proximally from the anterior approach by separating the brachioradialis and the brachialis from the lateral intermuscular septum.
9. The radial nerve is identified between the brachialis and brachioradialis. The posterior cutaneous nerve to the arm can then be released from the radial nerve, along with the posterior cutaneous nerve to the forearm.
10. The desired pedicle length is obtained by continuing dissection proximally while retracting the lateral head of the triceps posteriorly and the deltoid anteriorly. The pedicle is carefully dissected from the radial nerve while heading toward the spiral groove of the humerus. A small portion of the deltoid attachment to the humerus can be released to increase exposure.

    * An additional 6–8 cm of pedicle length can be obtained by splitting the lateral and long heads of the triceps and creating a tunnel underneath the triceps insertion. Of note, care must be taken to preserve the muscular branches to the triceps from the radial nerve in this technique [5].

    * Given the similar small diameters of the artery and vein, the authors often choose to mark the vein with an additional clip before harvest.
11. A single drain is placed. The donor site can typically be closed primarily with advancement flap closure and excision of standing cutaneous deformities.

Disclosure Statement No conflicts of interest to disclose.

References

1. Song R, Song Y, Yu Y, Song Y. The upper arm free flap. Clin Plast Surg. 1982;9(1):27–35.
2. Kang SY, Old MO, Teknos TN. Lateral arm free tissue transfer for parotid reconstruction: a pictorial essay. Head Neck. 2017;39(5):1015–9. https://doi.org/10.1002/hed.24695.
3. Rivet D, Buffet M, Martin D, et al. The lateral arm flap: an anatomic study. J Reconstr Microsurg. 1987;3(2):121–32. https://doi.org/10.1055/s-2007-1006974.
4. Urken M, Cheney M, Sullivan M, Biller H. Atlas of regional and free flaps for head and neck reconstruction. Raven Press; 1990.
5. Moffett TR, Madison SA, Derr JW Jr, Acland RD. An extended approach for the vascular pedicle of the lateral arm free flap. Plast Reconstr Surg. 1992;89(2):259–67. https://doi.org/10.1097/00006534-199202000-00010.
6. Katsaros J, Tan E, Zoltie N, Barton M, Venugopalsrinivasan V. Further experience with the lateral arm free flap. Plast Reconstr Surg. 1991;87(5):902–10. https://doi.org/10.1097/00006534-199105000-00015.

7. Brandt KE, Khouri RK. The lateral arm/proximal forearm flap. Plast Reconstr Surg. 1993;92(6):1137–43. https://doi.org/10.1097/00006534-199311000-00022.
8. Katsaros J, Schusterman M, Beppu M, Banis JC Jr, Acland RD. The lateral upper arm flap: anatomy and clinical applications. Ann Plast Surg. 1984;12(6):489–500. https://doi.org/10.1097/00000637-198406000-00001.
9. Martin D, Mondie JM, De Biscop J, Schott H, Peri G. The osteocutaneous outer arm flap. A new concept in microsurgical mandibular reconstructions. Rev Stomatol Chir Maxillofac. 1988;89(5):281–7. Le lambeau osteo-cutane brachial externe. Un nouveau concept dans les reconstructions mandibulaires microchirurgicales
10. Wolff K, Holzle F. Raising of microvascular flaps: a systematic approach. Springer; 2005.

Latissimus Dorsi Free Flap

23

Akash N. Naik and Avinash V. Mantravadi

History

- First described by Iginio Tansini in 1906 as a pedicled flap for use in breast reconstruction but did not gain popularity until the 1970s [1].
- Owens first utilized the pedicled latissimus for reconstruction of a head and neck oromandibular defect in 1955, but its application was widely expanded when first described as a free flap by Watson et al. in 1979 [2, 3].

Indications and Benefits

- Reconstruction of oral cavity, oropharynx, larynx, pharynx, cutaneous defects of the face/neck, skull base, and scalp defects.
  - Very useful for complex scalp/cranial reconstruction.
- Surface area of muscle and skin is large enough to accomplish total scalp reconstruction.
- Latissimus dorsi muscle is one of the thinnest muscles in the body with a large surface area. It is well vascularized with great versatility in combination with other flaps based off the subscapular system including "megaflap." [4]
- Can be used as a composite flap with separation of the cutaneous and muscular components when thoracodorsal artery perforator (TDAP) dissection is performed.
- Consistent and reliable vascular anatomy with regards to the thoracodorsal artery length and vessel caliber.
  - Average pedicle length of 9 cm when utilizing thoracodorsal artery alone (ranges from 5–16 cm) [5].
  - Pedicle length can be extended when dissection is carried up to include the subscapular artery.
  - 1.5–4 mm thoracodorsal artery diameter.
  - 2.5–4 mm venae comitans diameter.
- Minimal donor site morbidity from functional and cosmetic perspective.
- Can be harvested as muscle only, myocutaneous, or fasciocutaneous perforator flap with minimal muscle harvested.

A. N. Naik (✉)
Case Western Reserve University School of Medicine, Cleveland, OH, USA

MetroHealth Medical Center, Cleveland, OH, USA

A. V. Mantravadi
Department of Otolaryngology- Head and Neck Surgery, Indiana University School of Medicine, Indianapolis, IN, USA
e-mail: avmantra@iu.edu

R. Rezaee, A. Tamaki (eds.), *Local, Regional, and Free Flaps for Head and Neck Reconstruction*,
https://doi.org/10.1007/978-3-032-03211-9_23

Anatomy

- The latissimus dorsi muscle is a broad flat muscle covering a significant portion of the lower back from the iliac crest to the lower border of the scapula.
- The primary function of the latissimus is adduction, internal rotation, and extension of the arm; these muscular actions are well compensated by other muscles acting across the glenohumeral joint.
- Landmarks for the muscle:
  - Leading (anterior) edge can often be palpated on a line from the mid-axillary point to mid-point along the iliac crest between the anterior superior iliac spine (ASIS) and posterior superior iliac spine (PSIS).
  - In patients with larger body habitus, the humeral edge of the muscle can also be easily identified by horizontal abduction of the arm.
- The latissimus dorsi muscle can be divided into three primary angiosomes [6].
  - Proximal portion: supplied by thoracodorsal pedicle.
  - Mid and medial portion: supplied by posterior intercostal arteries.
  - Caudal portion: supplied by lumbar arteries.
    - The posterior intercostal and lumbar arteries are transected during the har vest. This may impact the reliability of the distal one-third of the muscle. This is important for consideration of the skin paddle design.
- Thoracodorsal vascular pedicle is a terminal branch of the subscapular system, which arises from the third portion of the axillary artery (Fig. 23.1).
  - Multiple branches arise from the thoracodorsal artery:
    - Muscular branches to subscapularis and teres major.
    - Angular branch to scapular tip.
    - Horizontal and vertical branches to the latissimus dorsi.
  - Pedicle typically inserts on the deep surface of the muscle approximately 8–10 cm inferior to the axilla.
  - After entering the muscle, divides into a vertical and horizontal branch that give off musculocutaneous perforators.
- The thoracodorsal nerve provides motor innervation to the latissimus dorsi muscle.
  - Arises from the posterior cord of the brachial plexus.
  - Typically runs between the artery and vein at the neurovascular hilum.
  - Approximately 8–19 cm can be harvested [5].

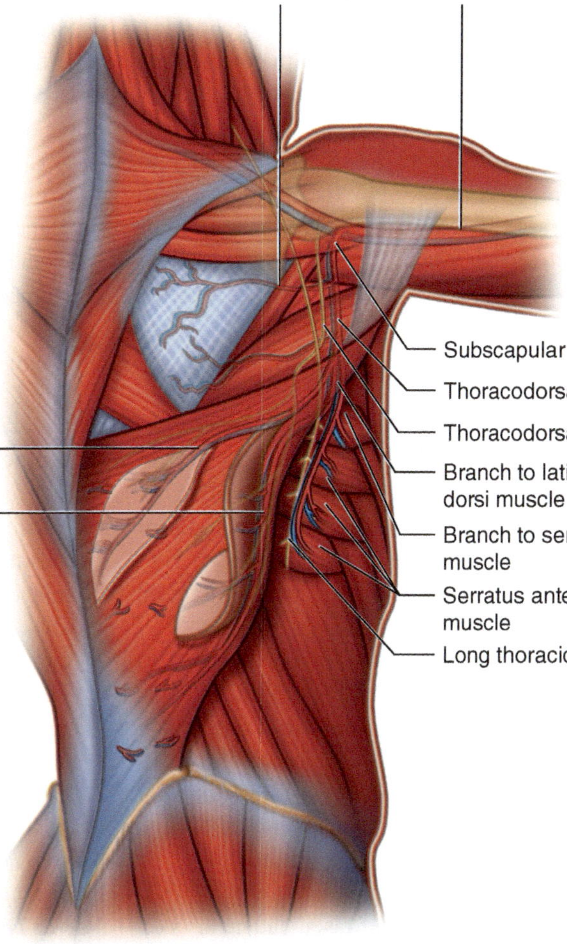

Fig. 23.1 Topographical anatomy of the latissimus free flap. It is supplied by the thoracodorsal artery and can be harvested as a myocutaneous, myofascial, or fasciocutaneous perforator flap. It is a highly versatile flap and can be utilized in combination with additional serratus muscle, parascapular/scapular skin, vascularized bone (rib, scapular tip, or lateral border), or thoracodorsal nerve

Preoperative Care

- Thorough evaluation of potential donor site including skin laxity, previous shoulder/back surgery, and thickness of subcutaneous tissue.
- Assess for history or scars from prior surgery or trauma that may compromise vascular anatomy and/or perfusion to the skin.
- Ensure patient understanding of hair-bearing skin considerations in setting of scalp/cranial reconstruction.
- Preoperative avoidance of intravenous or arterial lines in the surgical arm facilitates sterile preparation of the surgical site including the entire upper extremity.

Special Instruments and Positioning

- Flap can often be harvested with patient supine and arm positioned laterally or draped over chest/head/face without lateral positioning.
  - A limb positioner, mayo stand, or arm board can be helpful.
- Optional use of bean bag with patient placed in lateral decubitus position with axillary roll under contralateral arm.

  - Lateral decubitus positioning can be helpful when a large width of skin is harvested to facilitate closure of the donor site, or when flap is combined with others in the subscapular system.
- Prep the entire upper extremity and from mid-axillary line to ASIS and medially to the spine. Prep should extend anteriorly to the areola if wide flap elevation for donor site closure is required.

Modifications

- Can be harvested with additional muscle (serratus), skin (parascapular or scapular skin paddle), vascularized bone (rib, scapular tip, or lateral border), or nerve (thoracodorsal nerve, distal long thoracic nerve).
- Can be harvested as muscle only graft with subsequent skin grafting.
- Ability to harvest two separate myocutaneous skin paddles based off the horizontal and vertical branches of the thoracodorsal artery.
  - Chimeric skin paddles are particularly useful for reconstruction requiring external and intraoral skin paddles or for buried free flaps where monitoring may be difficult.
- TDAP allows harvest of fasciocutaneous skin paddle alone or with separate segment of muscle if two separate tissue types are required for defect. If TDAP to be used with latissimus, attention must be paid when designing skin paddle as perforators can be located anterior to the leading edge of the latissimus muscle and therefore injured during the deeper aspects of the skin incision along the muscle.
  - Modification in scalp/cranioplasty includes harvesting a broad area of muscle to cover the cranial defect to promote skin laxity and obliterate dead space for subsequent cranioplasty. Also, vital to reinforce thin scalp skin with muscle covering implant or hardware.
- Ability to be used as pedicled flap for head and neck reconstruction in vessel-depleted neck.

Pitfalls and Complications

- Positioning and two team harvest can be more difficult based on side of ablation.
- Risk of brachial plexus injury from positioning during harvest.
  - Likely secondary to impingement by the clavicle with exaggerated arm elevation [7].
- Higher potential for postoperative seromas given large volume of dead space after harvest and need for wide skin flap elevation.
- Risk of flap necrosis often due to skin paddle design extending to the far distal aspects.

Postoperative Care

- Physical therapy to help with range of motion and strengthening exercises early in postoperative course.
- Closed suction drains with removal based on surgeon preference and output.
- Optional abdominal binders to help prevent seroma, but not required.

Tissue type: *Myocutaneous, myofascial, or fasciocutaneous perforator flap*
Artery: *Thoracodorsal artery*
Vein: *Single venae comitans*
Nerve: *Thoracodorsal nerve*
Pedicle length: *5–16 cm*
Flap size: *up to 20 × 40 cm*

Operative Procedure

1. Design a curvilinear incision along the leading edge/anterior border of the latissimus dorsi.
   * Can be helpful to raise the arm over the head and pinch the posterior axillary fold (teres major and latissimus dorsi) and mark out the leading edge.
2. After skin incision, incise through subcutaneous tissue and identify the leading edge of the latissimus dorsi muscle and release the muscle from the loose areolar tissue anteriorly.
3. Important to skeletonize along the anterior edge of the latissimus from inferior to superior early

in dissection. Identify decussation between the serratus anterior muscle and latissimus as the flap is elevated off the chest wall.

* Care should be taken to stay directly on the muscle to prevent injury to the pedicle while working superiorly.

4. Identify the serratus branch on the superficial surface of the serratus muscle and trace back to the thoracodorsal artery. The thoracodorsal artery will insert deep to the latissimus humeral attachments (approximately 8–10 cm inferior to the axilla) (Fig. 23.1).
5. If harvesting skin, once the pedicle is identified, adjustments can be made to skin paddle design based on the geometry of pedicle and the amount and orientation of the needed tissue. Make posterior skin incision around skin paddle and dissect down to the latissimus muscle. Elevate skin flaps widely to expose latissimus muscle broadly.

   * Doppler is rarely needed due to extensive and robust network of perforators between the vertical and horizontal branches.
6. Transect distal and medial muscular attachments and bluntly dissect flap from chest wall as flap is elevated from distal to proximal.

   * If harvesting skin, care should be taken to compress the skin paddle and muscle together to avoid shearing of perforators.
7. As dissection continues superiorly, ligate the serratus anterior branch. If no bone is required, identify and ligate the angular branch as well.
8. Continueneurovascularpedicledissectionfrom distally to proximally. The thoracodorsal nerve will often be found between the artery and vein and will need to be ligated. With the pedicle clearly in view, divide the humeral attachments of the latissimus muscle.

   * Once these muscular attachments are divided, care should be taken to avoid traction injury to the vessels due to the weight of the flap.
9. If additional pedicle length is needed, continue dissection proximally and ligate the circumflex scapular artery to dissect out the subscapular artery.

   * The ability to manipulate the arm/shoulder with assistant or limb positioner greatly improves exposure during dissection of the proximal pedicle into the axilla.

   * Retractors, such as a Deaver or large Richardson, can be helpful with exposure based on body habitus and patient positioning.
10. After flap harvest, skin flaps are widely elevated in a suprafascial plane above the serratus and transected ends of the remaining latissimus muscle to facilitate primary closure. Multiple suction drains are typically required due to the large amount of dead space and wide elevation required for closure. They can be left in place for a longer than typical duration given the propensity for seroma collection.

Disclosure Statement No conflicts of interest to disclose.

References

1. Tansini I. Sopra il mio nuovo processo di amputazione della mammella (Italian). Riforma Med. 1906;12:757.
2. Owens N. A compound neck pedicle designed for the repair of massive facial defects: formation, development and application. Plast Reconstr Surg. 1946;1955(12):369–89.
3. Watson JS, Peter Craig RD, Orton CI. The free latissimus dorsi myocutaneous flap. Plast Reconstr Surg. 1979;64(3):299–305.
4. Aviv JE, Urken ML, Vickery C, Weinberg H, Buchbinder D, Biller HF. The combined latissimus Dorsi—scapular free flap in head and neck reconstruction. Archiv Otolaryngol Head Neck Surg. 1991;117(11):1242–50.
5. Urken ML, et al. Atlas of regional and free flaps for head and neck reconstruction: flap harvest and insetting. Lippincott Williams & Wilkins; 2012.
6. Taylor GI, Palmer JH. The vascular territories (angiosomes) of the body: experimental study and clinical applications. Br J Plast Surg. 1987;40(2):113–41.
7. Logan AM, Black MJ. Injury to the brachial plexus resulting from shoulder positioning during latissimus dorsi flap pedicle dissection. Br J Plast Surg. 1985;38(3):380–2.

24 Medial Sural Artery Perforator Free Flap

Andrew P. Katz and Kyle Mannion

History

- Most agree that the medial sural artery perforator (MSAP) free flap in its current form was introduced by Cavadas et al. in [1] with the use in head and neck reconstruction pioneered by Kao et al. in 2009 [2].

Indications and Benefits

- Best for reconstruction of oral cavity (tongue, lip, buccal mucosa), midface (maxillectomy and/or orbital exenteration), and cutaneous (cheek, ear) defects [3].
- Can also be used for pharynx and larynx reconstruction.
- Great alternative for patients in whom some bulk is required but the thickness of an anterolateral thigh free flap is too large due to body habitus.
  - Skin of posterosuperior calf is often thinner and less hair-bearing.
- Primary closure up to 6–7 cm width of donor site with low morbidity [4].

A. P. Katz (✉) · K. Mannion
Department of Otolaryngology- Head and Neck Surgery, Vanderbilt University Medical Center, Nashville, TN, USA
e-mail: kyle.mannion@vumc.org

Anatomy

- Medial sural artery branches off the popliteal artery near the femoral condyles. The vessel runs along the undersurface of the medial belly of the gastrocnemius muscle, and it branches into medial and lateral branches that perforate through the muscle to supply blood to the skin (Fig. 24.1) [3–6].
  - The medial sural artery is about 2 mm in diameter and pedicle length ranges from 9 to 16 cm based on the perforator used.
- The first perforator to the skin is typically 8 cm distal from the popliteal fossa crease in a line drawn from the middle of the crease to the medial malleolus, with additional perforators in the next distal 8 cm.
  - Perforators are typically 0.5–5 cm from the midline [3].
  - Perforators are about 1 mm in diameter [6].
- Venous drainage is from the venae comitantes. A superficial vein may also be present in the subcutaneous tissues superficial to the muscle that may be of larger caliber than the venae [3].
- Other vascular contributions to the muscle decreases the concern for muscle devascularization.

R. Rezaee, A. Tamaki (eds.), *Local, Regional, and Free Flaps for Head and Neck Reconstruction*,
https://doi.org/10.1007/978-3-032-03211-9_24

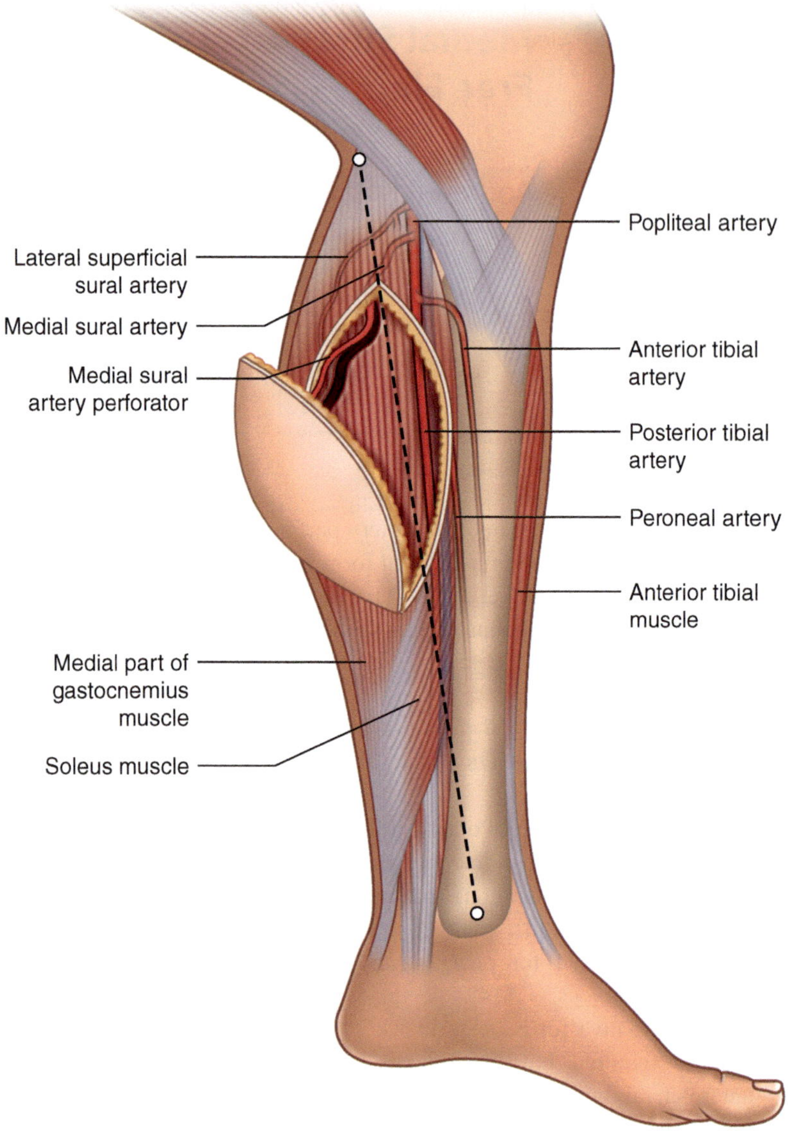

Fig. 24.1 The medial sural artery perforator flap can be a fasciocutaneous or musculocutaneous free flap. The skin is supplied by perforating branches of the medial sural artery, which runs within the gastrocnemius muscle. Perforators tend to pierce the gastrocnemius muscle to the skin along a line drawn from the middle of the popliteal crease to the medial malleolus

Preoperative Care

- Perform pinch test to determine width of skin paddle that can be taken that would still allow primary closure of the donor site.
- Evaluate thickness of the skin and subcutaneous tissue and determine if bulk is appropriate for reconstruction.

Special Instruments and Positioning

- Intraoperative positioning in a "frog-leg" position may ease harvest.
- Surgeon and assistant may approach from opposite sides of the leg.
- Optional use of tourniquet on thigh (300 mmHg).

  - Consider placing the tourniquet in a sterile fashion to allow a skin graft from the thigh if needed.

Modifications

- Can raise with plantaris tendon, or obtain via same incision, to use for resuspension of oral commissure [6].
- Saphenous or sural nerve can be raised for possible reinnervation.
- Split thickness skin graft can be used to close donor site if a larger skin paddle is needed and donor site cannot be closed primarily.
- Medial gastrocnemius muscle can be harvested to increase bulk [3, 6].

Pitfalls and Complications

- Literature reports that perforators to the skin are not identified in 5% of cases [3].
- Local skin necrosis at donor site has been seen in active smokers [3, 4].

Postoperative Care

- No postoperative limitations in weight-bearing.
- One closed suction drain with removal based on output.

Tissue type: *Fasciocutaneous, musculocutaneous*
Artery: *Medial sural artery*
Vein: *Venae comitantes*
Nerve: *Saphenous or sural nerve*
Pedicle length: *9–16 cm*[1–6]
Flap size: *Skin paddle length limited by length of lower leg, reports up to 14 cm. Width dependent on the patient and ability to close site primarily (recommended); although can use a split thickness skin graft and make skin paddle wide* [4, 5]

Operative Procedure

1. Perform a pinch test of the calf to estimate the maximum width of skin paddle that can be raised with the donor site closed primarily. Shave the leg as needed.
2. Draw a straight line between the middle of the popliteal crease and the medial malleolus. Use a handheld Doppler to identify skin perforators. The most proximal perforator will be approximately 8 cm below the popliteal crease with an additional 2–4 perforators in the subsequent 8 cm distal. Draw skin paddle centered along the identified perforators at the desired length and width (Fig. 24.1).
3. Prep the entire leg into the sterile field and drape appropriately.
   * Place padding around the thigh and an appropriately sized tourniquet (if desired) but not inflating until later in the harvest.
4. Position the leg in a "frog-leg" position to better visualize the posterior lower leg.
   * Cross-legged positioning has also been recently described [7].
5. Make the skin incision in the superior medial aspect of the skin paddle (the area where perforators are most likely to be clustered), and carry this down through the skin, fat, and gastrocnemius fascia to expose bare muscle. Carefully peel superficial gastrocnemius fascia laterally off the muscle and confirm that there are skin perforators.
6. Once the presence of perforators is confirmed, proceed with the remainder of the medial skin incision more distally and identify any additional perforators. Make a linear extension of the incision proximally toward the popliteal fossa to facilitate pedicle dissection later.
7. After perforators are identified, it may be useful to inflate the tourniquet. We recommend not inflating the tourniquet before perforator identification since the perforators are quite small and may be difficult to identify.

8. Gently retract the flap laterally and carefully trace each identified perforator through the gastrocnemius muscle to the medial sural artery. Trace and dissect the pedicle as proximally as necessary for pedicle length. The limit is the takeoff of the medial sural artery from the popliteal artery.

   * The artery caliber increases more proximally.
9. After pedicle dissection is complete, make the lateral incision of the skin paddle down to the gastrocnemius muscle to include skin perforators. At this time the flap should be completely free and attached to the body only by the pedicle.
10. Deflate the tourniquet. The flap can be harvested by ligating the medial sural artery and its venae comitantes.
11. Following the harvest, the donor site can be closed primarily with some additional undermining of the skin. If unable to close primarily, a split thickness skin graft can be used with an overlying bolster.

Disclosure Statement No conflicts of interest to disclose.

References

1. Cavadas PC, Sanz-Giménez-Rico JR, la Cámara AG, Navarro-Monzonís A, Soler-Nomdedeu S, Martinez-Soriano F. The medial sural artery perforator free flap. Plast Reconstr Surg. 2001;108(6):1609–15.
2. Kao HK, Chang KP, Chen YA, Wei FC, Cheng MH. Anatomical basis and versatile application of the free medial sural artery perforator flap for head and neck reconstruction. Plast Reconstr Surg. 2010;125(4):1135–45.
3. Hallock GG. The medial sural artery perforator flap: a historical trek from ignominious to "workhorse". Arch Plast Surg. 2022;49(2):240–52.
4. Cheng-Hung L, Hiseh YH, Lin CH. The medial sural artery perforator flap in lower extremity reconstruction. Clin Plastic Surgery. 2021;48:249–57.
5. Deek NFA, Hsiao JC, et al. The medial sural artery perforator flap: lessons learned from 200 consecutive cases. Plast Reconstr Surg. 2020;146(3):630–41.
6. Agrawal G, Chaudhary V, Choraria A, Dubey H. Medial sural artery perforator flap for head and neck reconstruction. Annals Maxillofac Sur. 2018;8(1):61–5.
7. Feng AL, Spector ME, Chinn SB, Holcomb AJ, Davies JC, Richmon JD, Lin DT, Varvares MA. Cross-legged modification for medial sural artery perforator flap harvest. Head Neck. 2023;45(3):752–6. https://doi.org/10.1002/hed.27263. Epub 2022 Dec 9. PMID: 36490216.

25 Omentum and Gastro-Omental Free Flap

Michael H. Berger and Eric M. Genden

History

- Free gastric flap was first described by Hiebert and Cummings in 1961 for reconstruction of the cervical esophagus [1], and free omentum flap was described by McLean and Buncke in 1972 for reconstruction of a scalp defect [2].
- The first composite gastro-omental flap is credited to Baudet in 1979 for closure of a pharyngostome [3].

Indications and Benefits

- Can be harvested as omentum only or a composite gastro-omental flap.
  - Gastro-omental flaps include a patch of gastric mucosa from the greater curvature of the stomach left in continuity with the greater omentum.
- In the head and neck, the omentum free flap has been reported for use in scalp wounds, neck wounds, hemifacial reconstruction, and anterior skull base osteomyelitis [4–7].
- The gastro-omental free flap is most commonly used for hypopharyngeal, laryngopharyngectomy, and esophageal reconstruction [8–14], but has been successfully utilized for reconstruction of oral cavity and oropharyngeal defects [9, 15].
  - Omentum can be harvested as a tube for pharyngoesophageal reconstruction.
- May be harvested as a free or pedicled flap, but uses of pedicled omentum in the head and neck are limited.
- Advantages of thin and pliable tissue, long pedicle, rich blood supply, and angiogenic and immunologic properties [16].
- Omentum has inherent healing, angiogenic, and immunologic properties advantageous for chronic wounds and in preventing wound breakdowns in patients treated previously with chemotherapy and/or radiation [4, 9, 17].
- Amenable to two-team approach [8].

Anatomy

- Omentum is a double layer of peritoneum that descends from the greater curvature of the stomach caudally as far as the pelvis, where it folds back on itself and attaches to the transverse colon, forming the gastrocolic ligament (Fig. 25.1) [18, 19].
- Dominant blood supply to the greater curvature of the stomach is derived from the right and left gastroepiploic arteries, which both are terminal branches of the celiac axis [20].

M. H. Berger · E. M. Genden (✉)
Department of Otolaryngology- Head and Neck Surgery, Icahn School of Medicine at Mount Sinai, New York, NY, USA
e-mail: eric.genden@mountsinai.org

R. Rezaee, A. Tamaki (eds.), *Local, Regional, and Free Flaps for Head and Neck Reconstruction*,
https://doi.org/10.1007/978-3-032-03211-9_25

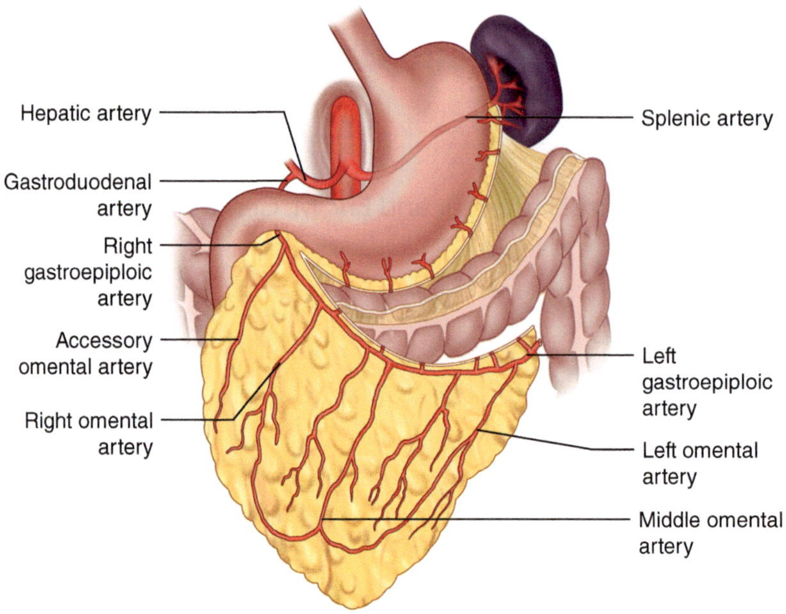

Fig. 25.1 The blood supply to the greater curvature of the stomach and omentum is demonstrated and is derived from the right and left gastroepiploic artery and vein. The flap can be pedicled on either the right or left gastroepiploic vessels, but the right gastroepiploic vessels are more commonly used. The flap can also be raised as omentum alone (as demonstrated pedicled on the right gastroepiploic artery) or as a composite gastro-omental flap, which includes a small patch of gastric mucosa from the greater curvature of the stomach

  - Right gastroepiploic artery branches from the gastroduodenal artery, which most commonly branches from the common hepatic artery (but may variably branch from the superior mesenteric artery or aorta).
  - Left gastroepiploic artery arises from the splenic artery.
- As the right and left gastroepiploic arteries course along the greater curvature of the stomach, they send off gastric branches to the stomach and omental branches to form the omental arterial arcade [4].
  - The omental arterial arcade has four major branches: right, middle, left, and accessory omental arteries.
  - There are rich anastomotic connections within the omental arcade, allowing for flexibility in flap design.
- Gastro-omental flap is equally supplied by the left and right gastroepiploic arteries and can be harvested based off either artery but right is often favored.
  - Right gastroepiploic vessels tend to have the dominant branches to the omentum and are larger caliber vessels, making them more suitable for microvascular anastomosis.
  - Harvest of the left gastroepiploic vessels carries increased risk for inadvertent splenic injury.

Preoperative Care

- Prior abdominal surgery and history of peritonitis would be relative contraindications due to scarring and adhesions in the abdominal cavity, causing the omentum to contract and making dissection more challenging.
- History of peptic ulcer disease can lead to acid production from transplanted tissue.

Special Instruments and Positioning

- Patient in supine position.
- General surgery team usually performs the intra-abdominal dissection.
- Gastrointestinal anastomosis stapler device for composite gastro-omental flap (not necessary for omental flap alone).
- Laparoscopic instruments if laparoscopic harvest to be performed.

Modifications

- May be harvested off either right or left gastroepiploic vessels.
- Can be harvested as omentum only flap or with patch of gastric mucosa in addition to omentum.
- Entire omentum may be harvested but can also harvest part of omentum based on branches of intra-abdominal arcade.
- Harvest of longer flap possible by utilizing gastric flap higher up along the greater curvature further away from pylorus.
- Laparoscopic harvest feasible and associated with reduced donor site morbidity [21].

Pitfalls and Complications

- Requires laparotomy or laparoscopy with risk of abdominal complications, including intra-abdominal abscess, abdominal hernia, gastrointestinal hemorrhage, gastric leak, and peritonitis.
- Gastric outlet obstruction (particularly if gastric mucosal portion of flap is harvested in close proximity to the pylorus).
- Potential for excess mucous production from flap.
- Potential for significant atrophy of flap.
- Cannot be raised with a skin paddle, so requires additional skin graft harvest should skin be required.

Postoperative Care

- Avoid heavy lifting for 6–8 weeks.
- May benefit from abdominal binder for 4 weeks.

Tissue type: *Visceral. Mucosa (from gastric portion) and adipose and lymphatic tissue (from omental portion)*
Artery: *Right gastroepiploic artery (primary), left gastroepiploic artery (secondary)*
Vein: *Right gastroepiploic vein (primary), left gastroepiploic vein (secondary)*
Nerve: *None*
Pedicle length: *20 cm (with range of 10–30 cm)* [9, 15, 22]
Flap size: *Average 25 × 35 cm (length × width) of omentum* [23]. *Mucosal graft from gastric antrum generally 8–14 cm long and 3–4 cm wide* [20]

Operative Procedure

Omentum Flap

1. Flap is harvested with patient in supine position.
2. Midline laparotomy incision is made cephalad to the umbilicus.
   * May also consider laparoscopic flap harvest [21].
3. Greater omentum is mobilized to the superior aspect of the abdomen allowing visualization of the avascular plane between the inferior aspect of the greater omentum and the transverse colon (Fig. 25.1).
   * Will frequently need to release intra-abdominal adhesions to effectively mobilize omentum.
4. Greater omentum is then released from its attachments to the transverse colon along its avascular plane. At this point, the omentum will be attached to the greater curvature of the stomach.

5. Omentum is then released from its gastrosplenic ligament, and the short gastric arteries branching from the gastroepiploic vessels are ligated.
6. Omentum is pedicled on both the right and left gastroepiploic arteries. The flap is most commonly based off the right gastroepiploic vessels given larger diameter; the left gastroepiploic artery is ligated just distal to its takeoff from the splenic artery.
7. Dissect the right gastroepiploic artery and vein to the pylorus and, when ready for harvest, ligate releasing the entire flap.

Gastro-Omental Flap

1. Initial steps are same as the omentum flap, with midline supra-umbilical laparotomy incision, followed by greater omentum mobilization and release of omentum from transverse colon attachments.
2. Identify the greater curvature of the stomach and mark out extent of gastric mucosa required for reconstruction.

   * Take care to ensure sufficient distance of gastric harvest away from pylorus to prevent gastric outlet obstruction.
3. Omental portion of the flap is vertically ligated along its orientation with gastric portion of the flap.
4. Divide the left gastroepiploic artery just distal to its takeoff from the splenic artery further mobilizing the flap. Stapler device used to divide gastric portion of the flap, beginning at the proximal end of the greater curvature toward the distal pyloric end. This will complete the mucosal harvest while simultaneously closing off the stomach.
5. Gastric mucosal graft will be in continuity with omentum, with flap now just pedicled on the right gastroepiploic artery, which can be dissected to the pylorus and then ligated to complete the flap harvest.

Disclosure Statement No conflicts of interest to disclose.

References

1. Hiebert CA, Cummings GO Jr. Successful replacement of the cervical esophagus by transplantation and revascularization of a free graft of gastric antrum. Ann Surg. 1961;154:103–6.
2. McLean DH, Buncke HJ. Autotransplant of the omentum to a large scalp defect. Plast Reconstr Surg. 1972;49(3):268–74.
3. Baudet J. Reconstruction of the pharyngeal wall by free transfer of the greater omentum and stomach. Int J Microsurg. 1979;1:53–9.
4. Mazzaferro D, Song P, Massand S, Mirmanesh M, Jaiswal R, Pu LLQ. The omental free flap-a review of usage and physiology. J Reconstr Microsurg. 2018;34(3):151–69.
5. Hultman CS, Carlson GW, Losken A, et al. Utility of the omentum in the reconstruction of complex extraperitoneal wounds and defects: donor-site complications in 135 patients from 1975 to 2000. Ann Surg. 2002;235(6):782–95.
6. Asai S, Kamei Y, Nishibori K, Katoh T, Torii S. Reconstruction of Romberg disease defects by omental flap. Ann Plast Surg. 2006;57(2):154–8.
7. Kokosis G, Vorstenbosch J, Lombardi A, et al. Use of the omental free flap for treatment of chronic anterior Skull Base infections. Plast Reconstr Surg – Glob Open. 2020:1–4.
8. Genden EM, Kaufman MR, Katz B, Vine A, Urken ML. Tubed gastro-omental free flap for pharyngoesophageal reconstruction. Arch Otolaryngol – Head Neck Surg. 2001;127(7):847–53.
9. Bayles SW, Hayden RE. Gastro-omental free flap reconstruction of the head and neck. Arch Facial Plast Surg. 2008;10(4):255–9.
10. Chahine KA, Chaffanjon P, Bettega G, Lebeau J, Reyt E, Righini CA. Gastro-omental free flap in the reconstruction of the unfavourable hypopharyngeal defects: a functional assessment. J Plast Reconstr Aesthetic Surg. 2009;62(11):1367–73.
11. Mixter RC, Rao VK, Katsaros J, Noon J, Tan E. Simultaneous reconstruction of cervical soft tissue and esophagus with a gastro-omental free flap. Plast Reconstr Surg. 1990;86(5):905–9.
12. Patel RS, Makitie AA, Goldstein DP, et al. Morbidity and functional outcomes following gastro-omental free flap reconstruction of circumferential pharyngeal defects. Head Neck. 2009;31(5):655–63.
13. Viñals JMV, Rodrigues TAG, Lopez CC, et al. Outcomes of gastro-omental free flap reconstruction for salvage Laryngopharyngectomy for pharyngeal and laryngeal cancer after concurrent Chemoradiotherapy. Ann Plast Surg. 2017;79(4):e20–4.
14. Righini CA, Bettega G, Lequeux T, Chaffanjeon P, Lebeau J, Reyt E. Use of tubed gastro-omental free flap for hypopharynx and cervical esophagus reconstruction after total laryngo-pharyngectomy. Eur Arch Oto-Rhino-Laryngol. 2005;262(5):362–7.

15. Gallagher J, Webb A, Ilankovan V. Gastro-omental free flaps in oral and oropharyngeal reconstruction: surgical anatomy, complications, outcomes. Br J Oral Maxillofac Surg. 2002;40(1):32–6.
16. Wei FC, Mardini S. Flaps and reconstructive surgery. Second ed. Elsevier; 2017.
17. Wang AW, Prieto JM, Cauvi DM, Bickler SW, De Maio A. The greater Omentum – a vibrant and enigmatic immunologic organ involved in injury and infection resolution. Shock. 2020;53(4):384–90.
18. Collins D, Hogan AM, O'Shea D, Winter DC. The omentum: anatomical, metabolic, and surgical aspects. J Gastrointest Surg. 2009;13(6):1138–46.
19. Di Nicola V. Omentum a powerful biological source in regenerative surgery. Regen Ther. 2019;11:182–91.
20. Urken ML. Atlas of regional and free flaps for head and neck reconstruction : flap harvest and insetting. 2nd ed. Philadelphia: Wolters Kluwer Health/ Lippincott Williams & Wilkins; 2012.
21. Craig SJ, Zhang A, Gardner TD, Clark JR, Ashford BG. Laparoscopic harvest of the gastro-omental free flap for reconstruction after total pharyngolaryngectomy: operative technique. Head Neck. 2017;39:1696–8.
22. Carlson GW, Thourani VH, Codner MA, Grist WJ. Free gastro-omental flap reconstruction of the complex, irradiated pharyngeal wound. Head Neck. 1997;19(1):68–71.
23. Das SK. The size of the human omentum and methods of lengthening it for transplantation. Br J Plast Surg. 1976;29(2):170–4.

26 Osteocutaneous Radial Forearm Free Flap

Melanie D. Hicks and Sarah L. Rohde

History

- The osteocutaneous radial forearm free flap (OCRFF) was first described by Song et al. in 1982 [1]. There was much excitement over its specific advantages including ease of harvest, long vascular pedicle, and a reliable skin paddle [2].
- However, in the late 1990s the OCRFF was no longer utilized as it once was due to studies reporting significant morbidity with pathologic radius fractures [3–5]. With the institution of prophylactic plating of the radius, the reduction in radius fractures regained popularity for the OCRFF [6].

Indications and Benefits

- Reconstruction of oral cavity, nasomaxillary complex, anterior maxillectomy, and palatal defects.
- Reliable flap with ease of harvest.
- Thin, well-vascularized, and pliable tissue with multiple uses.
- Long, reliable vascular pedicle.
  - Useful in patients with vessel-depleted neck, as the pedicle can reach the contralateral vessels [7].

Anatomy

- Lower arm arterial supply by the brachial artery divides into the radial and ulnar artery at the antecubital fossa.
- Radial artery terminates into the deep palmar arch (primarily supplies the first and second digit) and ulnar into the superficial palmar arch (primarily supplies the third, fourth, fifth, and part of second digit).
- Radial artery runs in the lateral intermuscular septum, which separates the flexor and extensor compartments of the forearm.
- Septocutaneous perforators are primarily located in the distal third of the forearm [8].
- Radial recurrent artery is the first major muscular branch from the radial artery and often viewed as the proximal limit of arterial pedicle harvest.
- Venous drainage is from the deep (two venae comitantes) and superficial (cephalic vein) systems (Fig. 26.1).
  - There are different branching patterns between these systems with variable degrees of communication [9].
  - Cephalic vein can be dissected through the upper arm to the subclavian vein for

M. D. Hicks (✉) · S. L. Rohde
Department of Otolaryngology- Head and Neck Surgery, Vanderbilt University Medical Center, Nashville, TN, USA
e-mail: s.rohde@vumc.org

R. Rezaee, A. Tamaki (eds.), *Local, Regional, and Free Flaps for Head and Neck Reconstruction*,
https://doi.org/10.1007/978-3-032-03211-9_26

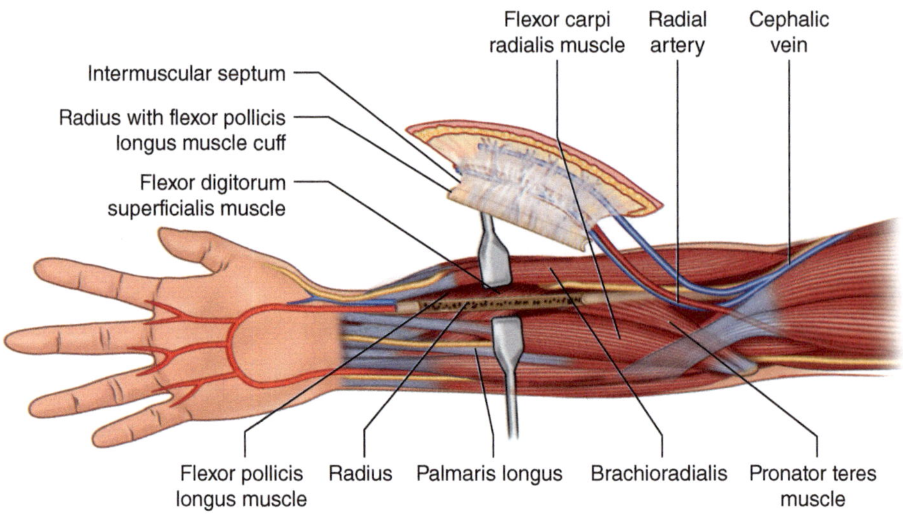

Fig. 26.1 Forearm anatomy demonstrating a raised osteocutaneous radial forearm free flap. The tissue and bone are perfused by the radial artery and venous drainage is through the vena comitantes and cephalic vein. The flexor digitorum superficialis is released from the radius and a cuff of flexor pollicis longus muscle is harvested along the bone. The pronator teres muscle mark the distal limits of available bone to harvest

additional length or even maintain flow by transposing and keeping pedicled [10].

- Innervation is supplied by the medial, lateral, and posterior antebrachial cutaneous nerves.
  - Lateral antebrachial cutaneous nerve runs with the cephalic vein and medial antebrachial cutaneous nerve with the basilic vein.
- Radial nerve is a mixed motor and sensory nerve.
  - Superficial branch of the radial nerve courses deep to the brachioradialis muscle, exits lateral to the tendon, and divides to provide sensation to the dorsum of the hand, and first, second, and third digits.
- The OCRFF is an extension of the RFFF whereby a partial thickness of the radius bone is harvested.
  - Perforating vessels from the radial artery to the periosteum perfuse the harvested radial bone.
  - Up to 12 cm length of the radius can be harvested.
  - Lateral retraction of the brachioradialis muscle tendon exposes the radial surface of the bone.
  - The flexor digitorum superficialis is released from the radius, exposing the flexor pollicis longus.
  - The flexor pollicis longus muscle attaches to the medial radius bone and is incised along the length of the bone, leaving a small cuff during harvest.
  - The pronator teres and pronator quadratus muscles classically mark the proximal and distal limits, respectively, of the available bone to harvest.
    - The pronator muscles can safely be released from the radius to provide a longer segment to harvest.
    - With use of a distal radius fracture plate, the quadratus muscle may also be split to increase the bony length.

Preoperative Care

- Allen's test assesses collateral blood flow to the hands from the ulnar artery with the radial artery occluded. The test identifies inadequate dual blood supply to the hand.
- Preoperative decision and protection on surgical arm (usually nondominant hand) to avoid placement of catheters and blood draws.

- Assess for history or scars from prior surgery or trauma that may compromise vascular anatomy or perfusion to the skin.
- Assess for history of traumatic injuries to the arm and previous surgeries to the radius. If uncertain, may obtain plain films.

Special Instruments and Positioning

- Optional use of tourniquet (250 mmHg, limit <2 h). Esmarch wrap can be used to exsanguinate the arm.
  - If torniquet is used, it is usually deflated for the bony portion of the harvest.
- Arm can be out on arm board and extended away from the operative bed for harvest.
- A fine-blade oscillating saw.
- Internal fixation instruments for radius defect.
  - 2.5–3.5 mm dynamic compression plate or long distal radius fracture plate.
  - Usually 8–14 hole plates are required.

Modifications

- Traditionally, the limit of bone harvest was defined by the pronator teres and pronator quadratus muscles. With an experienced surgeon, these muscles can be safely incised from the radius in order to increase the amount of bone that can be harvested.
- An extended bony harvest can be performed by sharply disinserting the brachioradialis tendon from the distal radius to gain access to the radial border and styloid tip [11].
- A keel shape modification can be implemented during bone harvest. Traditionally, this modification was believed to reduce donor-site fractures [12].
- One or two closing wedge osteotomies may be performed to create an anterior mandible or hemimandible.
- The double-barreled flap can provide adequate bone stock to support dental implants [13].

Pitfalls and Complications

- Radius fracture.
- Thin bone and lack of suitability for dental implants.
- Limited length of available bone when compared to the fibula, scapula, and iliac crest free flap.

Postoperative Care

- Apply bolster or wound vacuum on the forearm skin graft.
  - Dressing and bolster are generally removed within 5–7 days, but some may continue for longer.
- Apply volar splint from the midcarpal crease toward the elbow with wrist slightly extended.
- One closed suction drain with removal after 3–5 days based on output.
- Elevate splinted arm.
- Pulse oximeter on the ipsilateral thumb may reassure perfusion to the operative hand.
- Avoid weight-bearing activity of harvest arm for 6 weeks.

Tissue type: *Osteocutaneous*
Artery: *Radial artery*
Vein: *Cephalic vein, venae comitantes*
Nerve: *Antebrachial cutaneous nerve, superficial branch of the radial nerve*
Pedicle length: *14–22 cm*
Flap size: *Skin paddle from antecubital fossa to flexor crease. Maximum reported 35 × 15 cm. Harvestable bone reported to be maximum of 12 cm at 40–50% the diameter of the radius bone*

Operative Procedure

1. The skin flap is marked on the distal forearm, appreciating the location of the radial artery and cephalic vein. The distal skin paddle is

marked 2 cm proximal to the wrist crease to assist with skin coverage of the radius fixation hardware.

2. Skin incisions are made. We prefer to begin by incising around the skin paddle through subcutaneous fat. Radially, the cephalic vein is encountered and included in the flap elevation. The distal end of the cephalic vein will be ligated along with the lateral antebrachial cutaneous nerve (Fig. 26.1).
3. Dissection continues both from the radial and ulnar side until the flexor carpi radialis and brachioradialis muscle are encountered. Continue dissection in a subfascial plane, taking care to preserve the paratenon. The radial nerve will be seen as it emerges between the brachioradialis tendons. Care should be taken to preserve this nerve and exclude it from the fasciocutaneous flap.
4. The proximal incision is made from the antebrachial fossa to the skin flap incision distally. Particular attention to the cephalic vein is important, as it takes a more superficial path proximally. The cephalic vein is dissected free from the surrounding subcutaneous tissue.
5. Incise the lateral intermuscular septum between the brachioradialis and flexor carpi radialis muscle bellies in the proximal forearm to reveal the pedicle. The pedicle is freed from the proximal portion of the skin paddle to the antecubital fossa, taking care to clip any vessels off the pedicle.
6. The distal pedicle is ligated at the wrist.
7. The brachioradialis tendons are skeletonized. It is crucial to stay immediately on the tendon during this release, as incising too far from the tendon can shear perforators to the radius.
8. The flexor digitorum superficialis is separated from the pedicle.
9. The flexor pollicis longus muscle is then incised and freed from the radius, leaving a small cuff of muscle on bone.
10. The flexor pollicis longus is dissected off the radius until the pronator teres is encountered. This muscle can be dissected from the proximal radius to provide more bone length.
11. At this point, the pronator quadratus is encountered. It may be incised at the mid portion of the radius to provide additional length distally.
12. A beaver blade or similarly sharp instrument is used to demarcate the 40–50% diameter of the radius.
13. A fine-blade oscillating saw is used to make the bone cuts. The cut along the long axis of the radius should be no greater than 50% of the diameter of the radius to avoid radius fractures.
14. The vessels in the antecubital fossa are skeletonized to delineate the superficial and deep venous systems, as well as the artery.
15. Following the harvest, the radius is prophylactically plated with either a 2.5–3.5 mm dynamic compression plate or distal radius fracture plate depending on the preference of the surgeon and the length of the bony harvest.

    * Bicortical screws are employed.

    * Hand surgeons are consulted at many institutions for radial plating and are helpful in delineating the need for a distal radius fracture plate.
16. The arm is then closed. The flexor pollicis longus and brachioradialis tendon are sutured together to provide coverage of the hardware. The curvilinear incision is closed primarily, and the skin paddle defect can be closed with a full or split thickness skin graft (0.12–0.20 inch thickness). Bolster is placed and patient is placed in a volar splint.

Disclosure Statement No conflicts of interest to disclose.

References

1. Song R, Gao Y, Song Y, Yu Y, Song Y. The forearm flap. Clin Plast Surg. 1982;9(1):21–6.
2. Arganbright JM, Tsue TT, Girod DA, et al. Outcomes of the osteocutaneous radial forearm free flap for mandibular reconstruction. JAMA Otolaryngol Head Neck Surg. 2013;139(2):168–72. https://doi.org/10.1001/jamaoto.2013.1615.
3. Zenn MR, Hidalgo DA, Cordeiro PG, Shah JP, Strong EW, Kraus DH. Current role of the radial forearm free flap in mandibular reconstruction.

Plast Reconstr Surg. 1997;99(4):1012–7. https://doi.org/10.1097/00006534-199704000-00014.

4. Richardson D, Fisher SE, Vaughan ED, Brown JS. Radial forearm flap donor-site complications and morbidity: a prospective study. Plast Reconstr Surg. 1997;99(1):109–15. https://doi.org/10.1097/00006534-199701000-00017.
5. Thoma A, Khadaroo R, Grigenas O, et al. Oromandibular reconstruction with the radial-forearm osteocutaneous flap: experience with 60 consecutive cases. Plast Reconstr Surg. 1999;104(2):368–78; discussion 379–80. https://doi.org/10.1097/00006534-199908000-00007.
6. Bowers KW, Edmonds JL, Girod DA, Jayaraman G, Chua CP, Toby EB. Osteocutaneous radial forearm free flaps. The necessity of internal fixation of the donor-site defect to prevent pathological fracture. J Bone Joint Surg Am. 2000;82(5):694–704.
7. Rashid M, Tamimy MS, Masroor S, et al. Mandibular reconstruction using osteocutaneous radial forearm flap. J Coll Physicians Surg Pak. 2012;22(8):519–23.
8. Saint-Cyr M, Mujadzic M, Wong C, Hatef D, Lajoie AS, Rohrich RJ. The radial artery pedicle perforator flap: vascular analysis and clinical implications. Plast Reconstr Surg. 2010;125(5):1469–78. https://doi.org/10.1097/PRS.0b013e3181d511e7.
9. Thoma A, Archibald S, Jackson S, Young JE. Surgical patterns of venous drainage of the free forearm flap in head and neck reconstruction. Plast Reconstr Surg. 1994;93(1):54–9. https://doi.org/10.1097/00006534-199401000-00008.
10. Bhathena HM, Kavarana NM. Bipaddled, retrograde radial extended forearm flap with microarterial anastomosis for reconstruction in oral cancer. Br J Plast Surg. 1988;41(4):354–7. https://doi.org/10.1016/0007-1226(88)90072-0.
11. Matthews J, Ng W, Archibald S, Levis C. The use of the radial styloid in the extended osteocutaneous radial forearm free flap. Plast Surg (Oakv). 2016;24(2):89–95. https://doi.org/10.4172/plastic-surgery.1000967.
12. Weinzweig N, Jones NF, Shestak KC, Moon HK, Davies BW. Oromandibular reconstruction using a keel-shaped modification of the radial forearm osteocutaneous flap. Ann Plast Surg. 1994;33(4):359–69; discussion 369–70. https://doi.org/10.1097/00000637-199410000-00002.
13. Gonzalez-Castro J, Petrisor D, Ballard D, Wax MK. The double-barreled radial forearm osteocutaneous free flap. Laryngoscope. 2016;126(2):340–4. https://doi.org/10.1002/lary.25388.

Posterior Tibial Artery Free Flap

27

Alexandra E. Kejner

History

- First introduced in the literature by Zhang et al. in 1983 [1] in the Chinese literature and subsequently in the English language literature in 1984 [2].
- Described for head and neck reconstruction for the first time in 1991 by Chen et al. for total esophageal reconstruction [3].
- Interest rekindled for use in the head and neck in 2011 by Chan et al. using the posterior tibial artery free flap (PTAFF) for various sites in the head and neck including cutaneous reconstruction as well as intraoral lining [4].

Indications and Benefits

- Can be used for reconstruction of oral cavity, oropharynx, nasopharynx, larynx, pharynx, cutaneous, and skull base defects.
- Thin, well-vascularized, and pliable tissue with long pedicle and more easily concealed donor site.
- Consistent and reliable vascular anatomy
  - Long and large caliber pedicle up to 22 cm in length and 3 mm posterior tibial artery (PTA) diameter and 4 mm diameter vein [3, 4, 5].
- Skin paddle up to 30 × 15 cm^6 and slightly thicker than radial forearm but less subcutaneous tissue than anterolateral thigh flap [4].

Anatomy

- Arterial supply to the lower leg is from the posterior tibial, anterior tibial, and peroneal arteries (Fig. 27.1).
- The tibioperoneal trunk gives off the popliteal artery which branches to the PTA and anterior tibial artery (along with the posterior tibial nerve) where the terminal branches supply the foot [6].
- PTA arises at the border of the popliteus muscle between the tibia and fibula.
- PTA courses medially through the flexor compartment under the fibrinous arch of the soleus muscle and distally between the soleus and flexor digitorum longus muscles.
- PTA lays behind the tibia and the ankle joint. Proximally, the PTA is deep to the gastrocnemius, soleus, and deep transverse fascia. Distally, the vessels become superficial and just deep to the skin and fascia.

A. E. Kejner (✉)
Department of Otolaryngology- Head and Neck Surgery, Medical University of South Carolina, Charleston, SC, USA
e-mail: kejner@musc.edu

R. Rezaee, A. Tamaki (eds.), *Local, Regional, and Free Flaps for Head and Neck Reconstruction*,
https://doi.org/10.1007/978-3-032-03211-9_27

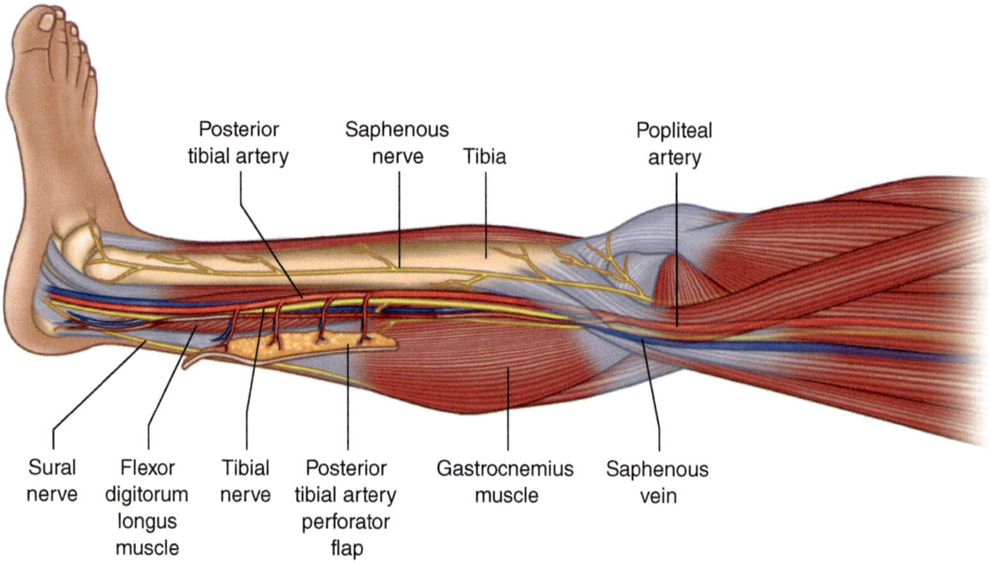

Fig. 27.1 Pertinent regional anatomy of the lower extremity of the posterior tibial artery free flap

- Typically, there are between one and four perforators with diameters between 0.4 and 2.1 mm (average 1.3 mm) [4].
- Venous drainage is provided by two venae comitantes creating the posterior tibial veins that travel with the PTA.
- The saphenous nerve is the terminal sensory branch of the femoral nerve, lies anterior to the long saphenous vein, and can be used in sensory innervation [1].

Preoperative Care

- Comparable to the preoperative work-up for fibula free flap harvest.
  - Computed tomographic angiography (CTA), magnetic resonance angiography (MRA), or color duplex Doppler ultrasonography (CDU) to assess for three-vessel runoff. CTA and MRA may more easily identify septocutaneous perforators for planning purposes [7].
- Patients with intractable diabetes or history of claudication may be better-suited for other donor sites due to concern for calcification of vessels as well as prolonged donor site healing [8].
- Avoid preoperative intravenous access to surgical leg.
- Take into consideration if patient may need a fibula free flap in the future and, if a possibility, consider alternate donor site.

Special Instruments and Positioning

- Optional use of tourniquet (250 to 300 mmHg, limit <2 h). Esmarch wrap can be used to further exsanguinate the leg.
  - Higher pressures may be needed in patients with hypertension or evidence of calcific disease of the vessels.
- Patient is positioned supine. The leg is then externally rotated with the leg straight and in a relaxed position. Avoid bending the leg as this can make the distal pedicle more difficult to visualize [8].
  - Leg can be left on the operative bed or alternatively onto an arm board if preferred.

Modifications

- An adipofascial extension can be harvested to provide additional tissue bulk and protective tissue around the pedicle and to minimize empty space in the resection cavity [9].
- Epidermis can be elevated off the flap to harvest just the deep fascia and subcutaneous tissue [10].
  - Epidermis can be closed primarily and avoid the need for skin grafting.
- Multiple perforators allow for the creation of separate perforator-based paddles [11].
- It can be raised as a dual-paddle skin flap without muscle, with the gastrocnemius muscle, or with the soleus muscle [11].
- Saphenous nerve is a sensory nerve that can be incorporated with the possibility of creating a sensate flap [1, 12].

Pitfalls and Complications

- Ischemic foot
- Poor take of donor site skin graft or prolonged healing (although risk of tendon exposure minimal due to donor site location)
- Sensory loss, pain, or paresthesia due to injury to saphenous nerve harvest or injury

Postoperative Care

- Apply negative pressure dressing or bolster on the skin graft.
  - While bolster is an option for this site, the author has found improved outcomes utilizing a wound vacuum for at least 1 week, with best outcomes at 2 weeks to facilitate mobilization without risk to skin graft.
- Boot or splint may be considered with a bolster.
- One closed suction drain with removal after 3 to 5 days based on output.
- Elevate leg when in bed. Ambulation can occur immediately.
- Compression stockings can assist in preventing edema of the foot.

Tissue type: *Adipofascial, fasciocutaneous*
Artery: *Posterior tibial artery*
Vein: *Posterior tibial vein (venae comitantes)*
Nerve: *Saphenous nerve*
Pedicle length: *7 to 25 cm*
Flap size: *Skin paddle along medial calf. Maximum reported 30 × 15 cm*

Operative Procedure

1. Patient is positioned supine with leg in relaxed position. The medial malleolus and medial patella are palpated and marked. The medial border of the tibia is palpated and marked as a reference point for the PTA. A handheld Doppler probe is used to identify skin perforators along the transverse intermuscular septum. The skin paddle is designed over the perforators oriented along the longitudinal axis of the PTA.
2. The anterior skin incision is made along the palpated medial border of the tibia and taken into the subfascial plane.
   * The tibia is identified by palpation only (avoid exposing the tibia).
3. Flexor digitorum longus muscular fascia is identified and reflected posteriorly. This will keep the tibia from becoming exposed by leaving the muscle in place and not disrupting the muscle tendon unit adjacent to the bone. This further allows for the identification of the septocutaneous perforators and PTA and venae comitantes in the septum between the flexor digitorum longus and soleus muscles.
   * At this time, the perforators that were previously identified can be seen arising from the main pedicle.

4. The posterior tibial nerve lays posterior to the pedicle and is dissected free from the vascular bundle.
5. The posterior skin is incised and extended into the subfascial plane overlying the soleus muscle.
6. The fascia is then reflected anteriorly, allowing identification of the previously identified perforators and vascular pedicle from the contralateral side.
7. The saphenous nerve and long saphenous vein are identified and preserved but can be included in the harvest.

   * Long saphenous vein harvest is not always necessary due to the caliber of the venae comitantes.
8. The posterior tibial artery and venae comitantes are ligated and divided at their distal aspect.

   * Recommend suture ligation or two medium clips due to potential for calcific changes to vessel which may make a single clip inadequate.
9. The superior aspect of the skin paddle is then incised, and the incision carried into the subfascial plane.
10. The flap is then elevated from distal to proximal, taking care to preserve the septocutaneous perforators. Muscular perforators are ligated and divided.
11. A vertical curvilinear incision along the medial aspect of the tibia can then be made as the flap is elevated along its pedicle.
12. The pedicle is then traced superiorly to its take-off from the tibioperoneal trunk.

   * The two venae comitantes do not tend to consolidate.
13. Following harvest, the donor site is closed. The superior aspect of the incision can be closed primarily. If no skin taken, this can be continued for the entirety of the leg. Otherwise, an appropriately sized skin graft can then be taken from the upper thigh or from the skin paddle of the PTAFF and secured with a negative pressure wound dressing.

   * Alternately, a full thickness or dermal substitute may be used.

Disclosure Statement No conflicts of interest to disclose.

References

1. Zhang SC. Clinical application of medial skin flap of leg--analysis of 9 cases. Zhonghua Wai Ke Za Zhi. 1983;21(12):743–5.
2. Okada T, Yasuda Y, Kitayama Y, Tsukada S. Salvage of an arm by means of a free cutaneous flap based on the posterior tibial artery. J Reconstr Microsurg. 1984;1(1):25–9. https://doi.org/10.1055/s-2007-1007050.
3. Chen HC, Tang YB, Noordhoff MS. Posterior tibial artery flap for reconstruction of the esophagus. Plast Reconstr Surg. 1991;88(6):980–6. https://doi.org/10.1097/00006534-199112000-00006.
4. Chan YW, Ng RWM, Wei WI. Anatomical study and clinical applications of free posterior tibial flap in the head and neck region. Plast Reconstr Surg. 2011;128(3):131e–9e. https://doi.org/10.1097/PRS.0b013e318221db67.
5. Mai L, Mashrah MA, Lin ZY, Yan LJ, Xie S, Pan C. Posterior tibial artery flap versus radial forearm flap in oral cavity reconstruction and donor site morbidity. Int J Oral Maxillofac Surg. 2022; https://doi.org/10.1016/j.ijom.2022.03.060.
6. Lezak B, Wehrle CJ, Summers S. Anatomy, bony pelvis and lower limb, posterior tibial artery. In: StatPearls; 2022.
7. Weng CRR, Thuener J, Zender C. Comparison of color flow Doppler, angiogram, CT angiogram and time resolved MR angiogram in the preoperative evaluation of lower extremity vascularity for fibular free flap reconstruction. J Otolaryngol Rhinol. 2016;2(011):1–5.
8. Kejner AE. The posterior tibial artery free flap for head and neck reconstruction. Curr Opin Otolaryngol Head Neck Surg. 2022;30(5):358–62. https://doi.org/10.1097/MOO.0000000000000843.
9. Mashrah MA, Mai L, Wan Q, et al. Posterior Tibial artery flap with an Adipofascial extension: clinical application in head and neck reconstruction with detailed insight into Septocutaneous perforators and donor-site morbidity. Plast Reconstr Surg. 2020;145(1):142e–52e. https://doi.org/10.1097/PRS.0000000000006396.
10. Ismail TI. The free fascial forearm flap. Microsurgery. 1989;10(3):155–60. https://doi.org/10.1002/micr.1920100302.
11. Mashrah MA, Mai L, Wan Q, Pan C. Chimeric posterior tibial artery flap: clinical application in oral and maxillofacial reconstruction. Int J Oral Maxillofac Surg. 2020;49(8):993–9. https://doi.org/10.1016/j.ijom.2019.12.008.
12. O'Connell DA, Reiger J, Dziegielewski PT, et al. Effect of lingual and hypoglossal nerve reconstruction on swallowing function in head and neck surgery: prospective functional outcomes study. J Otolaryngol Head Neck Surg. 2009;38(2):246–54.

Radial Forearm Free Flap

28

Akina Tamaki and Rod Rezaee

History

- First introduced in the Chinese literature by Yang et al. in 1981 [1] and further popularized beyond China for use in intraoral reconstruction [1, 2].

Indications and Benefits

- Reconstruction of oral cavity, oropharynx, larynx, pharynx, cutaneous, and skull base defects.
  - Useful in tubed laryngopharyngectomy defects.
- Thin, well-vascularized, and pliable tissue with multiple uses.
- Consistent and reliable vascular anatomy.
  - Long and large caliber pedicle up to 18 cm in length and 3 mm radial artery diameter [3]. The vein caliber will depend on the vein used and how proximally dissected.
- Large amount of forearm tissue from antecubital fossa to flexor crease can be harvested.

Anatomy

- Lower arm arterial supply by the brachial artery divides into the radial and ulnar artery at the antecubital fossa.
- Radial artery terminates into the deep palmar arch (primarily supplies the first and second digit) and ulnar into the superficial palmar arch (primarily supplies the third, fourth, fifth, and part of second digit).
- Radial artery runs in the lateral intermuscular septum, which separates the flexor and extensor compartments of the forearm.
- Septocutaneous perforators are primarily located in the distal third of the forearm [4].
- Radial recurrent artery is the first major muscular branch from the radial artery and often viewed as the proximal limit of arterial pedicle harvest.

A. Tamaki (✉)
Ear, Nose and Throat Institute, University Hospitals Cleveland Medical Center, Cleveland, OH, USA

Case Western Reserve University School of Medicine, Cleveland, OH, USA

Department of Otolaryngology- Head and Neck Surgery, Lewis Katz School of Medicine at Temple University, Philadelphia, PA, USA

R. Rezaee
Ear, Nose and Throat Institute, University Hospitals Cleveland Medical Center, Cleveland, OH, USA

Case Western Reserve University School of Medicine, Cleveland, OH, USA
e-mail: rod.rezaee@UHhospitals.org

R. Rezaee, A. Tamaki (eds.), *Local, Regional, and Free Flaps for Head and Neck Reconstruction*,
https://doi.org/10.1007/978-3-032-03211-9_28

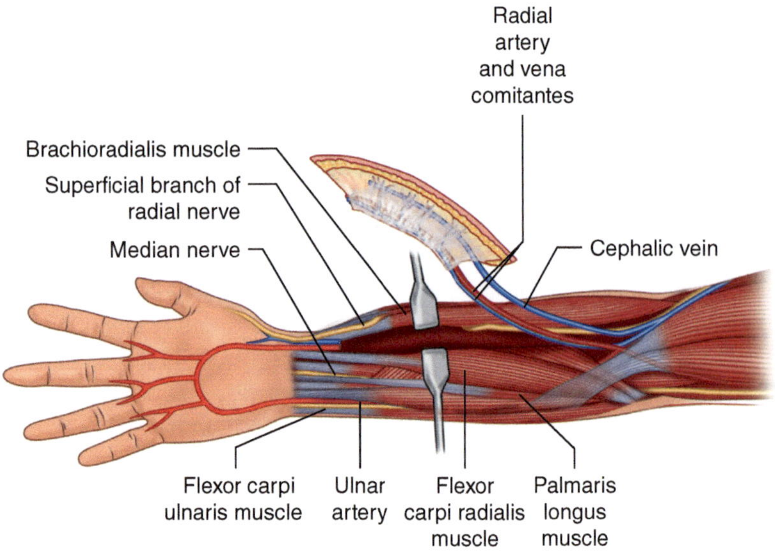

Fig. 28.1 Forearm anatomy demonstrating a raised radial forearm free flap. The tissue is perfused by the radial artery that courses between the flexor carpi radialis and brachioradialis muscle (retracted in this image). Venous drainage is through the vena comitantes and cephalic vein

- Venous drainage is from the deep (two venae comitantes) and superficial (cephalic vein) systems (Fig. 28.1).
  - There are different branching patterns between these systems with variable degrees of communication [5].
  - Cephalic vein can be dissected through the upper arm to the subclavian vein for additional length or even maintain flow by transposing and keeping pedicled [6].
- Innervation is supplied by the medial, lateral, and posterior antebrachial cutaneous nerves.
  - Lateral antebrachial cutaneous nerve runs with the cephalic vein and medial antebrachial cutaneous nerve with the basilic vein.
- Radial nerve is a mixed motor and sensory nerve.
  - Superficial branch of the radial nerve courses deep to the brachioradialis muscle, exits lateral to the tendon, and divides to provide sensation to the dorsum of the hand, and first, second, and third digits.

Preoperative Care

- Allen's test assesses collateral blood flow to the hands from the ulnar artery with the radial artery occluded. The test identifies inadequate dual blood supply to the hand.
  - Release of the ulnar artery should reperfuse the hand within 15 s.
  - Pulse oximeter attached to index finger or thumb can confirm findings. Occlusion of both ulnar and radial artery results in loss of the oximeter wave form. Then, release of the ulnar artery should result in return of the waveform.
  - Some centers advocate for vascular lab studies to assess for adequate ulnar flow.
- Preoperative decision and protection on surgical arm (usually nondominant hand) to avoid placement of catheters and blood draws.
- Assess for history or scars from prior surgery or trauma that may compromise vascular anatomy or perfusion to the skin.
- Skin tends to be thinner more distal on the forearm and in males. Skin often thicker on the radial aspect.
- Consider hair-bearing portions prior to harvest. The ulnar aspect of the flap is less hair-bearing.

Special Instruments and Positioning

- Optional use of tourniquet (250 mmHg, limit <2 h). Esmarch wrap can be used to exsanguinate the arm.
- Arm can be out on arm board and extended away from the operative bed for harvest.

Modifications

- Can be harvested with vascularized bone (radius), tendon (palmaris longus), nerve (antebrachial cutaneous nerve), or muscle (brachioradialis muscle).
- Epidermis can be elevated off the flap to harvest just the deep fascia and subcutaneous tissue [7].
  - The epidermis can be closed primarily and avoid the need for skin grafting.
- Separate skin islands and monitoring skin paddles can be designed.
  - Separate skin islands are particularly useful for laryngectomy defects or buried free flaps where monitoring may be difficult or an additional external skin defect is present [8].
- Beavertail modification with adipofascial extension of the proximal portion of the free flap [9].
  - This additional tissue can provide bulk or fill dead space (e.g., in total glossectomy, base of tongue, or maxillectomy defects).
- Full thickness skin grafts for donor site coverage can be harvested from the proximal forearm in small- to moderate-sized flaps and incorporated in the proximal incision near the antecubital fossa, if patient body habitus allows.

Pitfalls and Complications

- Ischemic hand.
- Poor take of donor site skin graft with possible risk of tendon exposure.
- Sensory loss, pain, or paresthesia due to injury to superficial branch of the radial nerve and transection of the antebrachial cutaneous nerve.

Postoperative Care

- Apply bolster or wound vacuum on the forearm skin graft.
  - Dressing and bolster are generally removed within 5–7 days, but some may continue for longer.
- Apply volar splint from the midcarpal crease toward the elbow with wrist slightly extended. May not need in setting of a wound vacuum.
- One closed suction drain with removal after 3–5 days based on output.
- Elevate splinted arm.
- Pulse oximeter on the ipsilateral thumb may reassure perfusion to the operative hand.

Tissue type: *Adipofascial, fasciocutaneous*
Artery: *Radial artery*
Vein: *Cephalic vein, venae comitantes*
Nerve: *Antebrachial cutaneous nerve, superficial branch of the radial nerve*
Pedicle length: *14–22 cm*
Flap size: *Skin paddle from antecubital fossa to flexor crease. Maximum reported 35 × 15 cm*

Operative Procedure

1. Plan a skin flap centered on the radial artery as well as a curvilinear incision to the antecubital fossa.
2. Skin incisions made. If starting with the curvilinear incision, identify the cephalic vein, which can be traced proximally and distally. Clip distal end of the cephalic vein as well as branches not draining the planned skin paddle. The lateral antebrachial cutaneous nerve has a close relationship with the cephalic vein and will need to be transected.

   * Care should be taken during incision at the distal (to avoid injuring branches of the radial nerve) and proximal skin incision (to avoid injuring cephalic vein).

   * Cephalic vein can be partially thrombosed in patients with prolonged hospitalizations and history of catheterization of the vein. The vein can be used proximal to the thrombosis or drainage can be based on the venae comitantes.

   * Lateral antebrachial cutaneous nerve along the cephalic can be harvested for an innervated flap.
3. Dissection can begin at the ulnar or radial aspect. On radial side, the brachioradialis muscle, cephalic vein, and superficial branches of the radial nerve are identified. On

the ulnar aspect, major landmarks include the palmaris longus and flexor carpi radialis. Dissect in the subfascial plane with careful preservation of the paratenon (Fig. 28.1).

* The superficial branch of the radial nerve can be readily found emerging between the brachioradialis tendon. All branches are dissected out of the flap toward the wrist.

* The palmaris longus can be harvested with the flap.

4. The brachioradialis and the flexor carpi radialis muscle and tendon are reflected to identify the radial artery and vena comitantes. Dissection continues from distally to proximally along the intramuscular septum with ligation of deeper branches suppling the forearm musculature and radius.

   * In the proximal forearm, the radial nerve will be found near the pedicle on the undersurface of the brachioradialis muscle.

5. The radial artery and vena comitantes pedicle can be traced up to the antecubital fossa to the branching point off the brachial artery. The radial recurrent artery (the first major branch off the radial artery supplying the muscle) may be identified and preserved. The venous anatomy should be carefully defined.

   * The two vena comitantes will often converge. The deep (vena comitantes) and superficial (cephalic vein) system will often also join but additional deeper veins will require ligation. Venous anastomosis can be based on either or both the deep and superficial systems [10].

6. Ligation of the distal radial artery and vena comitantes can be done earlier or at the end of the harvest.

   * If off tourniquet, intraoperative Allen test can be done to confirm adequate perfusion to the hand with the radial artery clamped.

7. Following harvest, the curvilinear incision is closed primarily, and the skin paddle defect can be closed with a full or split thickness skin graft (0.12–0.20 inch thickness). Bolster is placed and patient is placed in a volar splint.

   * Purse stringing of skin will decrease the size of the defect, but care must be taken not to overtighten.

   * Wound vacuums may be considered in patients with wound-healing concerns.

   * Other options include full thickness skin grafts (often from the ipsilateral forearm along the curvilinear incision to the antecubital fossa or upper arm) and transposition flaps (ulnar, rhomboid, bilobed).

Disclosure Statement No conflicts of interest to disclose.

References

1. Yang G, Chen B, Gao Y, Liu X, Li J, Jiang S, He S. Forearm free skin flap transplantation. Nat Med J China. 1981.
2. Soutar DS, Scheker LR, Tanner NS, McGregor IA. The radial forearm flap: a versatile method for intra-oral reconstruction. Br J Plast Surg. 1983;36(1):1–8. https://doi.org/10.1016/0007-1226(83)90002-4.
3. Cha YH, Nam W, Cha IH, Kim HJ. Revisiting radial forearm free flap for successful venous drainage. Maxillofac Plast Reconstr Surg. 2017;39(1):14. https://doi.org/10.1186/s40902-017-0110-8.
4. Saint-Cyr M, Mujadzic M, Wong C, Hatef D, Lajoie AS, Rohrich RJ. The radial artery pedicle perforator flap: vascular analysis and clinical implications. Plast Reconstr Surg. 2010;125(5):1469–78. https://doi.org/10.1097/PRS.0b013e3181d511e7.
5. Thoma A, Archibald S, Jackson S, Young JE. Surgical patterns of venous drainage of the free forearm flap in head and neck reconstruction. Plast Reconstr Surg. 1994;93(1):54–9. https://doi.org/10.1097/00006534-199401000-00008.
6. Bhathena HM, Kavarana NM. Bipaddled, retrograde radial extended forearm flap with microarterial anastomosis for reconstruction in oral cancer. Br J Plast Surg. 1988;41(4):354–7. https://doi.org/10.1016/0007-1226(88)90072-0.
7. Ismail TI. The free fascial forearm flap. Microsurgery. 1989;10(3):155–60. https://doi.org/10.1002/micr.1920100302.
8. Akin S, Basut O. A new flap design for monitoring the circulation of a buried free radial forearm flap in pharyngoesophageal reconstruction. J Reconstr Microsurg. 2002;18(7):591–4. https://doi.org/10.1055/s-2002-35097.
9. Seikaly H, Rieger J, O'Connell D, Ansari K, Alqahtani K, Harris J. Beavertail modification of the radial forearm free flap in base of tongue reconstruction: technique and functional outcomes. Head Neck. 2009;31(2):213–9. https://doi.org/10.1002/hed.20953.
10. Demirkan F, Wei FC, Lutz BS, Cher TS, Chen IH. Reliability of the venae comitantes in venous drainage of the free radial forearm flaps. Plast Reconstr Surg. 1998;102(5):1544–8. https://doi.org/10.1097/00006534-199810000-00030.

Rectus Abdominus Free Flap 29

Sara Yang, Sameep Kadakia, Yadranko Ducic, and Mark Wax

History

- First introduced in the literature by Brown et al. in 1975 [1].
- Described in head and neck reconstruction by Urken et al. in 1991 [2].
- Morbidity discussed by multiple authors [3–5].

Indications and Benefits

- Myocutaneous flap.
  - Reconstruction of high-volume soft tissue defects that benefit from myogenous and cutaneous components (e.g., skull base with orbital exenteration, lateral temporal bone, maxillectomy, sternal resections, and total glossectomy).
  - Myogenous component allows for obliteration of "dead spaces," while the cutaneous component allows for reconstruction of mucosal or cutaneous defects.
  - Cutaneous portion can reconstruct very large surface defects (25 × 25 cm).
- Myogenous flap.
  - Large soft tissue volume replacement for obliteration of large "dead spaces."
  - Separation of intracranial and extracranial components when there is a large defect such as for craniofacial resections or large volume maxillectomy defects.
- Perforator flaps.
  - Otherwise known as muscle-sparing rectus flaps or deep inferior epigastric perforator flaps (DIEP).
  - Can be utilized when the muscle component is not required.
  - Provides large soft tissue component with high volume adipose tissue (depending on anatomy), large surface area, and a long pedicle.
- Rectus abdominus muscle component is well defined in length and width.
- Fasciocutaneous portion can be harvested with large surface area but is variable in volume.
- Can be harvested as a two-team approach.
- Consistent and reliable vascular anatomy.
  - Long and large caliber pedicle 8–10 cm in length.
  - Inferior epigastric artery is consistently 3–4 mm with a 4–5 mm vein.

S. Yang (✉) · M. Wax
Department of Otolaryngology- Head and Neck Surgery, Oregon Health Sciences University, Portland, OR, USA
e-mail: waxm@ohsu.edu

S. Kadakia
Department of Surgery and Department of Plastic Surgery, Wright State University, Boonshoft School of Medicine, Dayton, OH, USA

Y. Ducic
Otolaryngology and Facial Plastic Surgery Associates, Fort Worth, TX, USA

R. Rezaee, A. Tamaki (eds.), *Local, Regional, and Free Flaps for Head and Neck Reconstruction*,
https://doi.org/10.1007/978-3-032-03211-9_29

Anatomy

- The internal iliac artery branches into the external iliac from which the inferior epigastric artery comes off (Fig. 29.1).
- The inferior epigastric vein empties into the external iliac, which then drains into the internal iliac vein.
- The vessels run together after exiting the lateral border of the muscle.
- The pedicle enters the lateral border of the muscle and runs deep to the muscle.
- Myocutaneous perforators are in the periumbilical region and are plentiful.
- The cutaneous portion in the contralateral periumbilical region can be harvested as the ipsilateral perforators supply a large watershed territory.
- The superior muscle is supplied by the superficial epigastric pedicle. This vessel needs to be ligated when harvesting the flap. The muscle remains viable based on the inferior vessels.
- Venous drainage is from the deep veins that accompany the perforating arteries.
  - These veins form two venae comitantes that accompany the artery. These vessels consistently join to form one large vein 2–3 cm from the external iliac vein.
- Innervation is supplied by multiple branches entering the lateral aspect of the muscle. These are easily identified and divided.

Preoperative Care

- Abdomen is examined for scars or evidence of abdominal surgery.
  - Midline laparotomy, Pfannenstiel, appendectomy, enteral feeding tube, and inguinal hernia scars must be considered when selecting this as a flap donor site but are not an absolute contraindication.
  - Umbilical hernias or evidence of paramedian hernia following laparotomy is a rela-

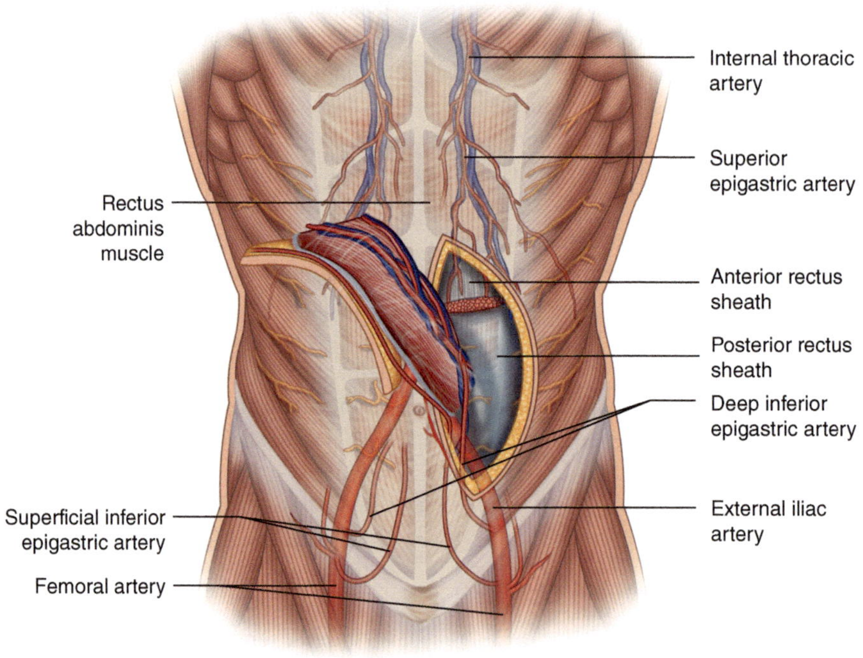

Fig. 29.1 Rectus abdominis free flap clinical anatomy. The adipofascial tissue and rectus abdominis muscle is pedicled on the deep inferior epigastric vessels

tive contraindication and a different flap should be considered.
- When composite tissue is required, the quantity of adipose tissue present needs to be assessed. It can be quite bulky.
- Adipose tissue is not an issue when only the myogenous portion is to be harvested.
- In multiparous women the perforators may be anatomically inconsistent.
- Recommend using side opposite enteral feeding tubes or prior scars.

Special Instruments and Positioning

- Drape from the bottom of the costal margin to the pubis and lateral to the anterior iliac crest bilaterally.
- A set of large and deep retractors depending on the body habitus should be available.

Modifications

- Can be harvested as a myogenous flap, myocutaneous flap, or perforator cutaneous flap.
- DIEP flap harvest or transverse rectus abdominus muscle (TRAM) have been well described in breast reconstructive surgery.
- Due to variability of angiosomes, the use of infrared perfusion technology may help define areas of marginal vascularity, especially in flaps with large or obliquely oriented cutaneous paddles.
- Skin and facia should be harvested above the arcuate line to maintain the integrity of the fascial closure.
- Consideration for reinforcing the abdominal closure.

Pitfalls and Complications

- Significant adipose tissue can make dissection of the pedicle tedious.
- Need to be familiar with abdominal wall closure.
- Hernia is rare and reported to be <3%.
- Retroperitoneal hematomas are infrequent but can occur.
- Dissection must be careful below the arcuate line to minimize chance of inadvertent violation of the peritoneal cavity.
- Potential for postoperative atelectasis and ileus.
- Rarely the artery may be involved by atherosclerotic disease and require more technical expertise.
- Skin color match is poor for cutaneous defects in the head and neck.

Postoperative Care

- Apply abdominal binder for 1 week and then for patient comfort as needed.
- Two closed suction drains with removal after 3–5 days based on output.
- Incentive spirometry with respiratory therapy consult to prevent atelectasis.
- Early mobilization with no restrictions.

Tissue type: *Adipocutaneous, myocutaneous, myogenous*
Artery: *Deep inferior epigastric artery*
Vein: *Deep inferior epigastric vein*
Nerve: *segmental mixed motor/sensory has been described via the lower six intercostal nerves*
Pedicle length: *8–10 cm*
Flap size: *Muscle is variable in length depending on body height. Width is usually 8 cm. The adipose tissue volume is variable based on body habitus. Most of the skin of the abdominal wall can be harvested. Flaps up to 25 × 25 cm have been described*

Operative Procedure

1. Mark the following external anatomical measures:
   (a) *Linea alba in the midline*: This will help define the midline and most medial aspect of the anterior rectus sheath.
   (b) *Arcuate line*, a line from one anterior superior iliac crest to the contralateral.

This marks the point where, inferior to the line, the posterior rectus sheath is no longer present. Reconstruction of the anterior sheath either primarily or with tissue reinforcement is necessary to prevent bulging and hernia formation. Design modification and anterior sheath preservation below the arcuate line aids in primary closure of this area.

(c) A line drawn vertical from the anterior superior iliac crest to the ribcage. Another line drawn midway between this line and the linea alba. This marks the lateral border of the rectus muscle.

2. Plan the cutaneous component centered on the periumbilical perforators. They can extend across the midline if needed. Leave the umbilicus as is. The skin paddle can be shaped as desired to fill the defect. It should be positioned to allow primary skin closure.
3. Skin incisions are made through the dermis with a sharp blade. Dissection is then done with cautery to the level of the anterior sheath. Starting lateral, the subcutaneous tissue is dissected medially until the skin perforators are seen coming through the anterior sheath. At this point the anterior sheath is incised just lateral to the perforators with care being taken not to sheer them. The sheath is then cut around the skin paddle on the ipsilateral side of the skin paddle. The skin paddle on the contralateral side is freed from the fascia to the midline.

   * If not needed for the reconstruction (i.e., dural or skull base repair or for soft tissue suspension), only the portion of the rectus sheath in the region around the perforator need be harvested. This preservation of the anterior rectus fascia will aid in primary closure of the sheath after harvest.
4. The skin incision is then extended superiorly to below the costal cartilage. The anterior sheath is divided and the rectus muscle is freed from the anterior sheath superiorly and inferiorly being careful to leave the skin paddle attached to the rectus sheath through which its perforators flow. Only a portion of the rectus sheath around the preserved perforators need be included (Fig. 29.1).
5. The dermis is tacked to the rectus muscle to prevent shearing of the skin paddle while the flap is being manipulated.
6. Once the rectus muscle has been identified anteriorly and by its medial and lateral borders, it is freed up by blunt dissection from the posterior rectus sheath above the arcuate line. The superior attachment to the costal cartilages is divided and the muscle is reflected inferiorly. Near the arcuate line the vascular pedicle is easily identified and followed inferiorly to where it exits the lateral aspect of the muscle and from here travels inferolaterally into the pelvis as it approaches the external iliac system. It is necessary to divide the lateral muscular aponeurosis to maximize pedicle length and expose the inferior aspect of the rectus muscle if needed for bulk.

   * Care must be taken to repair the anterior sheath below the arcuate line where the posterior sheath is absent. Careful dissection must be followed to minimize chance of violating the peritoneal cavity in this area.

   * The vascular pedicle lies in fibro fatty tissue and is easily isolated and followed inferiorly to the external iliac vessels. The two venae comitantes will combine into a single vein before entering the external iliac vein. These vessels are ligated when it is time to transfer the flap.

   * Wide malleables placed posterior to the pedicle protect the abdominal contents and facilitate the dissection by keeping the fatty contents out of view while larger retractors (e.g., Deaver or Richardson retractors) can be beneficial as well to aid the lower dissection of the pedicle to its origin.
7. The tendinous insertions that run perpendicular to the muscle can be stuck to the anterior sheath and require slower and more meticulous dissection. The rectus muscle above the proximal most insertion may have its vascularity dependent on the superior epigastric vessels and not be amenable to inclusion in the flap.

8. The flap is now attached inferiorly to the pubic bone and by its vascular pedicle. The inferior attachment to the pubic bone is divided and the pedicle is dissected. The pedicle is ligated and the flap transferred to the head and neck region when the ablation is complete.
9. Closure of the donor site starts with the anterior rectus sheath. Our preference is to start superiorly and use a running large nonabsorbable suture. Many methods are described and seem to be institution specific. All report excellent closure. Closure of the site where the skin has been removed depends on the amount of anterior rectus sheath removed. Many times, with small volume cutaneous paddles, the anterior sheath can be closed using the same suture in a primary fashion. Consider using a malleable to protect violating the posterior rectus sheath and to facilitate suturing. Drains are placed above this layer and the skin and subcutaneous tissues are closed in multiple layers of absorbable sutures.

   * If there is any tension, reinforcement with mesh or allogenic substances should be utilized [6]. Many have been described and are again institutionally dependent.

   * An abdominal binder is utilized for 7 days.

Disclosure Statement No conflicts of interest to disclose.

References

1. Brown RG, Vasconez LO, Jurkiewicz MJ. Transverse abdominal flaps and the deep epigastric arcade. Plast Reconstr Surg. 1975;55(4):416–21. PMID: 123346. Wanamaker JR, Burkey BB. Overview of the rectus abdominis myocutaneous flap in head and neck reconstruction. Facial Plast Surg 1996 12(1):45–50. https://doi.org/10.1055/s-2008-1064492. PMID: 9244007.
2. Urken ML, Turk JB, Weinberg H, Vickery C, Biller HF. The rectus abdominis free flap in head and neck reconstruction. Arch Otolaryngol Head Neck Surg. 1991;117(8):857–66. https://doi.org/10.1001/archotol.1991.01870200051007. PMID: 1654058
3. Lo JO, Weber SM, Andersen PE, Gross ND, Gosselin M, Wax MK. Atelectasis after free rectus transfer and abdominal wall reconstruction. Head Neck 2008 30(10):1339–1343.https://doi.org/10.1002/hed.20880. PMID: 18720521.
4. Reece MK, Langenfeld TL, Pak KY, Wax MK, Tan K, Slijepcevic A, Petrisor D, Alwani M, Johnson RM, Ducic Y, Kadakia SP. Impact of smoking on donor site following rectus flap harvest for head and neck reconstruction. Am J Otolaryngol 2023 44(4):103847. https://doi.org/10.1016/j.amjoto.2023.103847. Epub 2023 Mar 20. PMID: 36989752.
5. Houdek MT, Bakri K, Tibbo ME, Wagner ER, Rose PS, Sim FH, Moran SL. Outcome and complications following vertical rectus abdominis myocutaneous flap surgery to reconstruct sacrectomy defects. Plast Reconstr Surg. 2018;142(5):1327–35. https://doi.org/10.1097/PRS.0000000000004890.
6. Saman M, Kadakia S, Ducic Y. Does the use of an acellular dermal graft in abdominal closure after rectus flap harvest impact the occurrence of post-operative hernia? Oral Maxillofac Surg. 2015;19(4):347–51. https://doi.org/10.1007/s10006-015-0498-1. Epub 2015 Apr 26. PMID: 25910994.

30 Scapular and Parascapular Free Flaps

Janice L. Farlow and Amit Agrawal

History

- Initial anatomical studies of the subscapular system was described by Saijo in 1978 [1] with subsequent surgical reports of the scapular flap by Dos Santos in 1980 [2] and the parascapular flap by Nassif in 1982 [3].

Indications and Benefits

- Reconstruction of various soft tissue and/or bony defects of the head and neck.
  - Can be combined with scapular bone, rib, or latissimus/serratus muscle as a chimeric free flap for complex defect reconstructions of multiple tissue types.
  - Large defects can be resurfaced by combining a scapular and parascapular flap [4].
- Good color match to facial skin and often non-hair-bearing.
- Reliable primary closure of donor site up to a flap width of 8–10 cm.
- Consistent landmarks for the circumflex scapular artery (CSA).
- Generally, the subscapular arterial system has less atherosclerotic disease than the lower extremities [5].

Anatomy

- Both the scapular and parascapular flaps are supplied by the CSA (Fig. 30.1).
  - Most often, the CSA branches 1–4 cm from the origin of the subscapular artery, which arises from the distal third of the axillary artery.
  - In 3–20% of patients, the CSA can arise directly off of the axillary artery [6–8].
- The CSA is identified in the triangular space, which is bounded by the teres major inferiorly, teres minor superiorly, and the long head of the triceps laterally.
  - The CSA has two main branches—a deep periosteal branch running underneath the teres major to supply the scapular bone, and a superficial branch.
- The superficial branch divides into a transverse and a descending branch, which supply the scapular and parascapular flaps, respec-

** Please see the Scapular Tip and Lateral Scapular Border Free Flap chapter on details of harvesting bone from the subscapular system.*

J. L. Farlow (✉)
Department of Otolaryngology- Head and Neck Surgery, Indiana University, Indianapolis, IN, USA

A. Agrawal (✉)
Department of Otolaryngology- Head and Neck Surgery, The James Cancer Hospital and Solove Research Institute, The Ohio State University, Columbus, OH, USA
e-mail: amit.agrawal@osumc.edu

R. Rezaee, A. Tamaki (eds.), *Local, Regional, and Free Flaps for Head and Neck Reconstruction*,
https://doi.org/10.1007/978-3-032-03211-9_30

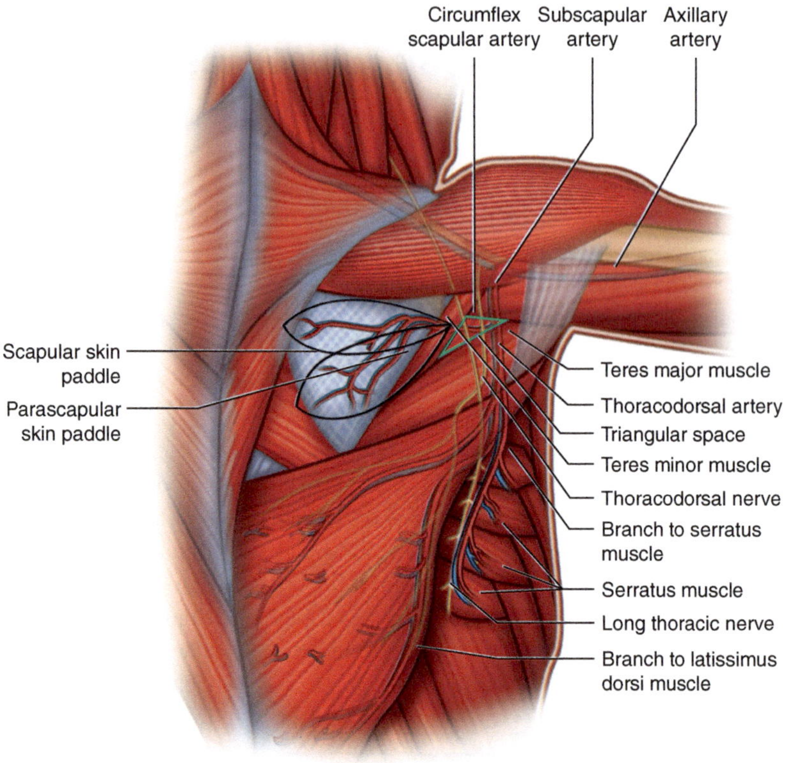

Fig. 30.1 The subscapular arterial system is depicted, with the circumflex scapular artery seen emanating from the triangular space (green triangle: bounded by the long head of the triceps brachii, teres minor, and teres major muscles) to supply the scapular and parascapular skin paddles. The subscapular arterial system continues separately as the thoracodorsal artery, which supplies the serratus and latissimus dorsi muscles

tively. Each paddle can be up to 25–30 cm, with a width of 8–10 cm to allow for primary closure.
  - The scapular and parascapular paddles are often combined for larger flaps [4]. Some have also reported that multiple skin paddles may be harvested only connected by the dorsal thoracic fascia, allowing separation between the cutaneous paddles [9].
- The length of the pedicle is increased by carrying the dissection proximally. Taking the transverse or descending branches of the CSA at its origin creates a pedicle length of 4–6 cm.
- If the CSA alone is taken, its proximal diameter is 1–4 mm, for a pedicle length of 7–10 cm [10]. If you ligate the other branches of the subscapular vessels, the pedicle can be lengthened to 11–14 cm with a 3–8 mm proximal diameter of the subscapular artery [11].
- Venous drainage consists of two venae comitantes of the CSA between 2.5 and 4 mm in diameter [10]. The venae either join with the thoracodorsal vein (90%) or enter the axillary vein separately (10%) [2].
- The dorsal rami of the spinal nerves supply cutaneous innervation to the region. No reports of a successful sensate parascapular flap have been reported despite attempts [12].

Preoperative Care

- A thorough history and examination for scars should be performed of the axilla and shoulder girdle to determine if prior surgery (e.g., axillary lymph node dissection) or trauma may compromise the vascular supply to the flap.

Special Instruments and Positioning

- The flap can be harvested in the supine, lateral decubitus, or prone positions.
- The shoulder, back, lateral thorax, and upper arm should be circumferentially prepped to

allow for intraoperative movement of the arm to facilitate vessel identification. A beanbag [13] or just an arm board [14] can be used to support the decubitus or supine positions.
  - An intraoperative assistant [15], Mayo stand [14], or specialty arm bed attachment [13] can be used to assist with arm mobilization intraoperatively.
- Ensure that all pressure points are padded and that the patient is well supported if in the lateral decubitus position. If a Mayo stand or specialty arm attachment is used, a stockinette can be used to aid in padding and positioning.
- If adjusting the position of the arm intraoperatively, be sure to avoid excessive external rotation of the shoulder to avoid brachial plexus injuries.

Modifications

- Composite flaps can include vascularized bone (lateral scapular border, scapular tip, and/or rib) or muscle (teres major or teres minor off muscular branches from the CSA; or latissimus and/or serratus from the thoracodorsal artery).
- The flap can be de-epithelialized to create an adipofascial flap. Additionally, the thickness of the flap can be reliably adjusted down to the level of the dorsal thoracic fascia in situations where there is too much tissue bulk for appropriate inset.
- If a larger cutaneous paddle is desired, the scapular and parascapular flaps can be combined [4].

Pitfalls and Complications

- Difficulty raising the flap simultaneously with the ablative procedure given positioning.
- Shorter pedicle length, particularly if the flap is harvested from the posterior triangle approach.
- Possibility of shoulder dysfunction, although reportedly low even with harvest of the scapular bone [11, 16].
  - Excessive external rotation of the shoulder can also lead to brachial plexopathies.
- Widened scars are common on the upper back, particularly if large paddles are harvested.

Postoperative Care

- For cutaneous paddles alone, general limitation of heavy lifting and routine incision care are all that is required.
- If muscle and/or bone is taken as a composite flap, consider immobilization of the arm for 3–4 days postoperatively.
- Postoperative physical therapy is important to restore range of motion and strength of the shoulder girdle over time.

Tissue type: *Adipofascial, fasciocutaneous*
Artery: *Circumflex scapular artery*
Vein: *Venae comitantes or circumflex scapular vein*
Nerve: *None*
Pedicle length: *Variable depending on extent of dissection, range from 4 to 14 cm*
Flap size: *Maximum of 10 × 30 cm*

Operative Procedure

1. The cutaneous paddle is designed either horizontally (antero-posteriorly) over the superior third of the scapula for the scapular flap, or vertically (cranio-caudally) over the lateral scapula bone for the parascapular flap. For either flap, it is mandatory to incorporate the triangular space.

   * Doppler can be used preoperatively to identify the location of the CSA in the triangular space, particularly in obese patients where the fossa is not easily palpated.
2. Elevate flap distal to proximal in the layer superficial to the deep muscular fascia of the back. Just before reaching the triangular space, the fascia is incised and elevated with the flap (Fig. 30.1).
3. Once the pedicle is exposed, the proximal skin incision can be completed, with elevation toward the pedicle.

4. The pedicle can then be traced into the triangular space.

   * The parascapular artery has been reported to appear in the subcutaneous tissues between the teres major and the superior border of the latissimus dorsi muscle. When this happens, the teres major must be divided to pass the pedicle through [17].

5. Depending on desired pedicle length, dissect into the triangular space and divide branches to the teres minor and the scapular bone (this branch must be preserved for lateral scapula border bone flaps). If the patient has a subscapular artery and no additional flap components from the thoracodorsal artery, the thoracodorsal branch can be taken at its origin to gain an extra centimeter of pedicle length and possibly a larger vessel.

   * The teres major muscle can be divided to drop the pedicle into the axilla if needed, with re-approximation of the muscle after the flap is harvested. If there is concern for devascularization of the teres major, some advocate avoiding reattachment to avoid additional fibrosis and resultant shoulder dysfunction [18].

   * If approaching from the posterior aspect, a counter incision in the axilla can be performed to aid in visualization [19].

6. The donor site can typically be closed primarily.

Disclosure Statement No conflicts of interest to disclose.

References

1. Saijo M. The vascular territories of the dorsal trunk: a reappraisal for potential flap donor sites. Br J Plast Surg. 1978;31(3):200–4. https://doi.org/10.1016/s0007-1226(78)90082-6.
2. dos Santos LF. The vascular anatomy and dissection of the free scapular flap. Plast Reconstr Surg. 1984;73(4):599–604. https://doi.org/10.1097/00006534-198404000-00014.
3. Nassif TM, Vidal L, Bovet JL, Baudet J. The parascapular flap: a new cutaneous microsurgical free flap. Plast Reconstr Surg. 1982;69(4):591–600. https://doi.org/10.1097/00006534-198204000-00001.
4. Koshima I, Soeda S. Repair of a wide defect of the lower leg with the combined scapular and parascapular flap. Br J Plast Surg. 1985;38(4):518–21. https://doi.org/10.1016/0007-1226(85)90013-x.
5. Dowthwaite SA, Theurer J, Belzile M, et al. Comparison of fibular and scapular osseous free flaps for oromandibular reconstruction: a patient-centered approach to flap selection. JAMA Otolaryngol Head Neck Surg. 2013;139(3):285–92. https://doi.org/10.1001/jamaoto.2013.1802.
6. Senturk S, Efe D, Ozkan A, Goncu RG, Zumrut M. Multidetector computed tomography angiography to evaluate the subscapular arterial tree. Microsurgery. 2015;35(8):640–4. https://doi.org/10.1002/micr.22499.
7. Valnicek SM, Mosher M, Hopkins JK, Rockwell WB. The subscapular arterial tree as a source of microvascular arterial grafts. Plast Reconstr Surg. 2004;113(7):2001–5. https://doi.org/10.1097/01.prs.0000122235.09892.da.
8. Barrett TF, Orlowski H, Rich J, Jackson RS, Pipkorn P, Puram SV. Anatomic variants of the subscapular-thoracodorsal arterial system: a radiologic analysis of 200 arterial systems. Oral Oncol. 2022;125:105682. https://doi.org/10.1016/j.oraloncology.2021.105682.
9. Thoma A, Archibald S, Payk I, Young JE. The free medial scapular osteofasciocutaneous flap for head and neck reconstruction. Br J Plast Surg. 1991;44(7):477–82. https://doi.org/10.1016/0007-1226(91)90001-z.
10. Wolff K, Holzle F. Raising of microvascular flaps: a systematic approach. Springer; 2005.
11. Urken M, Cheney M, Sullivan M, Biller H. Atlas of regional and free flaps for head and neck reconstruction. Raven Press; 1990.
12. Upton J, Albin RE, Mulliken JB, Murray JE. The use of scapular and parascapular flaps for cheek reconstruction. Plast Reconstr Surg. 1992;90(6):959–71. https://doi.org/10.1097/00006534-199212000-00003.
13. Stevens JR, Rosko AJ, Marchiano E, et al. The spider limb positioner in subscapular system free flaps. Oral Oncol. 2018;85:24–8. https://doi.org/10.1016/j.oraloncology.2018.08.004.
14. Eskander A, Kang SY, Ozer E, et al. Supine positioning for the subscapular system of flaps: a pictorial essay. Head Neck. 2018;40(5):1068–72. https://doi.org/10.1002/hed.25051.
15. Nishimura T, Furukawa M, Koshima I. Scapular bone flap harvests of patients in a supine position. Laryngoscope. 2004;114(6):1130–2. https://doi.org/10.1097/00005537-200406000-00033.
16. Coleman SC, Burkey BB, Day TA, et al. Increasing use of the scapula osteocutaneous free flap. Laryngoscope. 2000;110(9):1419–24. https://doi.org/10.1097/00005537-200009000-00001.
17. Wei F-C, Mardini S. Flaps and reconstructive surgery. Elsevier; 2009.
18. Blackwell K, Cheney M, Harris J, Hadlock T. Atlas of regional and free flaps for head and neck reconstruction. Lippincott Williams & Wilkins; 2011.
19. Gahhos FN, Tross RB, Salomon JC. Scapular free-flap dissection made easier. Plast Reconstr Surg. 1985;75(1):115–8. https://doi.org/10.1097/00006534-198501000-00027.

31 Scapular Tip and Lateral Scapular Border Free Flap

Catherine Haring

History

- Osteocutaneous scapular free flaps based off of the subscapular vascular system were first described in the 1980s [1–3].
- In the 1990s, it was reported that the scapular tip could be harvested independently from the lateral border [4].

Indications and Benefits

- Used for boney defects of the mandible, maxilla, or orbit or in defects requiring composite tissue reconstruction with bone and soft tissue.
- Ideal flap in patients with vascular disease of the lower extremity.
- When harvested as a chimeric flap, each component is supplied by a separate artery and vein, allowing for mobility of soft tissue components relative to bone.
- The scapular tip is triangular and can be harvested in a variety of three-dimensional shapes [5].
- Periosteal blood supply allows for osteotomies when needed.

C. Haring (✉)
Department of Otolaryngology- Head and Neck Surgery, The Ohio State University, Columbus, OH, USA
e-mail: Catherine.haring@osumc.edu

- Reliable vascular anatomy.
  - Pedicle length:
    - 4–14 cm for circumflex scapular artery-based lateral scapular border [6].
    - Up to 20 cm for angular artery-based scapular tip [5].
  - Absence of atherosclerosis of vessels, which can be seen in distal extremities [7].
- When harvested in a supine position, can be harvested in two-team approach [8, 9].
- Minimal functional morbidity at the donor site.

Anatomy

- Arterial supply is based on the subscapular artery, which is a branch of the axillary artery (Fig. 31.1).
  - The subscapular artery gives off the circumflex scapular and thoracodorsal arteries as its main branches.
  - The subscapular artery gives off the circumflex scapular artery, which passes through the triangular space (formed by teres major, teres minor, and long head of triceps muscle).
  - The circumflex scapular artery divides into a descending periosteal branch supplying the lateral scapular border and a superficial circumflex scapular artery supplying the skin. The skin branch divides into a trans-

R. Rezaee, A. Tamaki (eds.), *Local, Regional, and Free Flaps for Head and Neck Reconstruction*,
https://doi.org/10.1007/978-3-032-03211-9_31

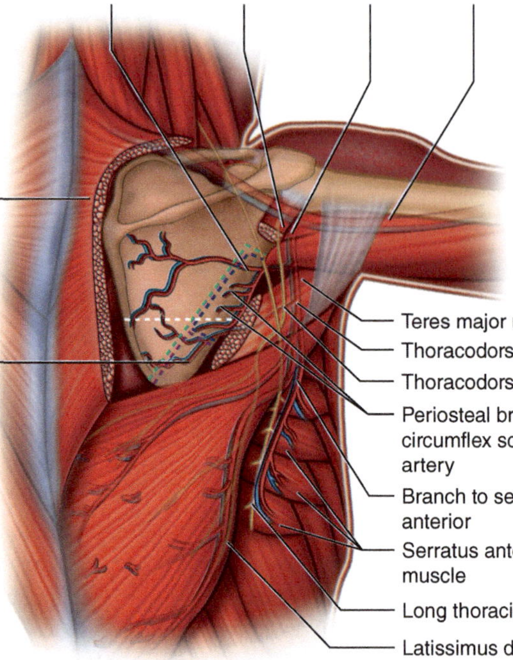

Fig. 31.1 Anatomy of the scapular tip and lateral scapular border free flap (right posterior scapula). The vascular supply of the scapular free flaps is based on the subscapular artery and vein. The subscapular artery gives of the circumflex scapular artery, which passes through the triangular space, and the thoracodorsal artery. The thoracodorsal artery travels ventral to the teres major muscle and gives of the serratus anterior artery, angular artery, and terminates in the latissimus muscle. An osseous scapular flap can be harvested based off the angular artery/vein (scapular tip free flap, white and purple dotted lines) or off the circumflex scapular artery/vein (lateral scapular border, blue dotted line) or off both vascular branches (green dotted line)

verse/horizontal branch and a descending cutaneous branch from which scapular and parascapular fasciocutaneous flaps are harvested.

  - The thoracodorsal artery gives off the serratus anterior artery and angular arteries and terminates in the latissimus dorsi muscle. The branch into the latissimus muscle divides into horizontal and vertical branches.
  - The branch points for the serratus, angular, and latissimus arteries can be variable, but most commonly branch close to one another, creating a trifurcation.
- Venous drainage is from accompanying veins of the same name.
- Sensory innervation is from intercostal nerves. There is no single nerve that innervates a large region and therefore cannot be used as a sensitized flap.
- Motor innervation is provided by the thoracodorsal and long thoracic nerves.
  - Thoracodorsal nerve supplies motor innervation to the latissimus muscle and is divided when muscle is harvested with the flap.
  - Long thoracic nerve supplies motor innervation to serratus anterior muscle and is divided when muscle is harvested with flap.
- Numerous extrinsic and intrinsic muscles are harvested or require transection for this flap.
  - Extrinsic muscles:
    - Latissimus muscle originates from the thoracic vertebra and inserts onto the humerus.

  - Serratus anterior muscle originates from ribs and inserts along the medial and inferior angle of the scapula.
- Intrinsic muscles:
  - Subscapularis lies on anterior (ventral) surface of the scapula.
  - Infraspinatus lies on posterior (dorsal) surface of the scapula.
  - Teres major originates from posterior scapular tip and inserts onto humerus.
  - Teres minor originates from posterior lateral border of scapula and inserts onto humerus.

Preoperative Care

- Preoperative decision and protection of surgical arm (usually nondominant hand) to avoid placement of catheters.
- Assess for prior history of axillary dissection (e.g., breast cancer surgery or shoulder replacement).
- Obese patients may have considerably thick subcutaneous tissue.
- No special studies are required prior to operation.

Special Instruments and Positioning

- Can be harvested in a supine position, semi-decubitus position, lateral position or prone.
- The supine/semi-decubitus position allows for a two-team approach and will be described below.
- When harvested in a supine position, a limb positioner, mayo stand, or arm board can be helpful [8, 10].

Modifications

- Can be harvested with vascularized bone (scapular tip, lateral border, rib), muscle (latissimus dorsi, serratus anterior), and/or skin (scapular, parascapular, thoracodorsal artery perforator).
- If a skin paddle is needed when harvesting the scapular tip, the latissimus muscle/skin paddle or thoracodorsal artery perforator is most commonly used.
- If a skin paddle is needed when harvesting the lateral scapular border, the parascapular or scapular skin paddles are most commonly used.
- Both the scapular border and scapular tip can be harvested, either as one long segment of bone or as two independently vascularized bone segments, along with several soft tissue components as listed above. In some circumstances or based on specific defect needs, the serratus muscle can be harvested with a segment of rib.
- There is no sensory nerve, but motor nerves (thoracodorsal and long thoracic nerves) can be harvested when latissimus or serratus are harvested.
  - These nerves and branches can be harvested and used as cable grafts or can be anastomosed into donor motor nerves in the ablative site to, theoretically, maintain muscle bulk in situations that may potentially be beneficial (e.g., into the hypoglossal nerve in the setting of a total glossectomy).

Pitfalls and Complications

- Rarely, the circumflex scapular artery and thoracodorsal artery can branch directly and separately off of the axillary artery, resulting in an absent subscapular artery and the need for multiple anastomoses [11].
- When harvested as a chimeric flap, care must be taken during inset to ensure proper geometry of the vessels associated with each component as torsion may occur.

Postoperative Care

- Closed suction drains are placed in the wound. Often one drain remains in place at discharge as serosanguinous drainage can occur for prolonged periods of time.

- Within several days following surgery, range of motion exercises are started. Physical therapy is used after discharge when needed. Full shoulder function is typically regained within 1 month.

Tissue type: *Fasciocutaneous, myofascial, osseous*
Artery: *Subscapular artery*
Vein: *Subscapular vein*
Nerve: *Thoracodorsal and long thoracic nerves*
Pedicle length: *4–14 cm for circumflex scapular artery-based lateral scapular border, up to 20 cm for angular artery-based scapular tip flap*
Flap size: *10–14 cm of bone length for scapular artery-based lateral scapular border, 6–9 cm for angular artery-based scapular tip*

Operative Procedure

The following steps describe the procedure as observed from an anterior perspective when the patient is positioned in a supine or semi-decubitus position.

Angular Artery-Based Scapular Tip

1. An incision is created along the anterior leading edge of the latissimus dorsi muscle.
   * Modification of this incision must be considered if a TDAP flap is being considered due to the perforators potentially not traveling through the lateral aspect of the muscle.
2. The latissimus dorsi muscle is retracted posteriorly, identifying the intermuscular space between the chest wall/serratus anterior muscle bellies and the latissimus dorsi muscle.
3. Blunt dissection is performed within the intermuscular space, and the vascular pedicle is identified. This includes the thoracodorsal artery along with the branches to the serratus anterior muscle, angular artery, and terminal vessels within the latissimus muscle (Fig. 31.1).
   * Doppler can be helpful to locate the pedicle or a component of the pedicle in those with large amounts of subcutaneous tissue.
4. The angular artery branch is clearly delineated originating from the thoracodorsal artery or serratus branch and terminating on the anterior surface of the scapular tip.
5. If separate soft tissue components are needed, these are harvested at this time. Most commonly, this includes harvesting the latissimus dorsi muscle with or without overlying skin. If separate soft tissue components are not needed, the serratus and latissimus vascular branches are ligated and divided.
6. The serratus anterior muscle attachments along the inferior scapular tip are divided, allowing for lateral retraction of the scapular tip away from the chest wall.
7. The thoracodorsal artery pedicle is traced as it travels under the teres major muscle toward the axilla.
8. The teres major muscle attachments along the posterior border of the scapular tip are divided, taking care to protect the vascular pedicle.
9. Divide the subscapularis muscle along the anterior and infraspinatus on the posterior surface of the scapula at site of planned osteotomies.
10. Osteotomies are created and remaining muscle attachments are divided.
11. Vascular pedicle is traced superiorly until the circumflex scapular artery and vein are encountered.
    * If pedicle length is needed, the circumflex scapular branches are ligated and divided.
12. Following harvest, the cut teres major muscle is reattached to the remnant scapular bone. Closed suction drains are placed in the wound and the donor site incision can be closed primarily.

Circumflex Scapular Artery-Based Lateral Scapular Border

1. A scapular or parascapular skin paddle is designed overlying the lateral scapular border encompassing the triangular fossa. The triangular fossa is located in the space

between the long head of the triceps muscle and the teres major and minor muscles. A vertically oriented skin paddle is easier to harvest in the supine/semi-decubitus position (Fig. 31.1).

* The location of the triangular fossa can be approximated with the use of the Doppler traveling up the lateral border until the vessels are heard as the circumflex scapular exits the space.

2. The skin incision is made and deepened through the skin and subcutaneous fat until the posterior border of the latissimus dorsi muscle is encountered. The posterior border latissimus muscle is reflected anteriorly off the scapular tip and lower aspects of the lateral border, revealing the teres major muscle. The lateral scapular border can be palpated.
3. Subfascial dissection is performed along the posterior border of the teres major muscle until the superficial circumflex scapular artery/vein supplying the skin is identified.
4. Blunt dissection is performed over the pedicle into the triangular fossa.
5. When soft tissue is required, posterior skin incision is made to harvest the parascapular/scapular skin paddle, ensuring inclusion of the cutaneous vascular pedicle that was previously identified. Subfascial dissection is performed, releasing the skin paddle off of the deltoid, triceps, and teres minor muscles.

   * Doppler can be useful in identifying the circumflex scapular artery as it exits the triangular fossa and can be mapped into the transverse/horizontal branch and descending branches. This can aid in designing the skin paddle when needed.
6. The teres minor and major muscles are divided, revealing the lateral scapular border and descending periosteal branch of the circumflex scapular artery/vein.

   * Remnant teres muscle attached to the scapular tip can be thinned as needed to reduce muscle bulk.
7. If the scapular tip is harvested in continuity with the lateral scapular border, the serratus attachments to the tip are divided, allowing lateral retraction of the scapula away from the chest wall.
8. If separate soft tissue components are not needed, the serratus and latissimus vascular branches are ligated and divided, taking care to leave the angular artery intact if the tip is harvested with the flap. If the tip is not harvested, the thoracodorsal artery/vein can be ligated and divided after the take-off of the circumflex scapular artery/vein. If the latissimus and serratus muscles are not harvested, the respective nerves can be carefully preserved.
9. At the site of planned osteotomies, the subscapularis muscle is divided along the anterior surface of the scapula and the infraspinatus muscle is divided along the posterior surface of the scapula. Division of remaining muscle attachments is typically done after the osteotomy if body habitus prevents sufficient retraction of the scapula away from the thorax.
10. Osteotomies are created.
11. The vascular pedicle is traced superiorly until the take-off from the axillary artery/vein. Closed suction drains are placed in the wound and the donor site incision can be closed primarily. Closed suction drains are placed in the wound and the donor site incision can be closed primarily.
12. Following harvest, the cut teres major muscle is reattached to the remnant scapular bone. Closed suction drains are placed in the wound and the donor site incision can be closed primarily.

    * Drill holes can be used to assist with securing the teres major muscle to the bone if sufficient soft tissue is not present.

Disclosure Statement No conflicts of interest to disclose.

References

1. dos Santos LF. The vascular anatomy and dissection of the free scapular flap. Plast Reconstr Surg. 1984;73(4):599–604. https://doi.org/10.1097/00006534-198404000-00014.

2. Gilbert A, Teot L. The free scapular flap. Plast Reconstr Surg. 1982;69(4):601–4. https://doi.org/10.1097/00006534-198204000-00002.
3. Swartz WM, Banis JC, Newton ED, Ramasastry SS, Jones NF, Acland R. The osteocutaneous scapular flap for mandibular and maxillary reconstruction. Plast Reconstr Surg. 1986;77(4):530–45. https://doi.org/10.1097/00006534-198604000-00003.
4. Coleman JJ, Sultan MR. The bipedicled osteocutaneous scapula flap: a new subscapular system free flap. Plast Reconstr Surg. 1991;87(4):682–92. https://doi.org/10.1097/00006534-199104000-00013.
5. Chepeha DB, Khariwala SS, Chanowski EJP, et al. Thoracodorsal artery scapular tip autogenous transplant: vascularized bone with a long pedicle and flexible soft tissue. Arch Otolaryngol Head Neck Surg. 2010;136(10):958–64. https://doi.org/10.1001/archoto.2010.166.
6. Gibber MJ, Clain JB, Jacobson AS, et al. Subscapular system of flaps: an 8-year experience with 105 patients. Head Neck. 2015;37(8):1200–6. https://doi.org/10.1002/hed.23738.
7. Yoo J, Dowthwaite SA, Fung K, Franklin J, Nichols A. A new angle to mandibular reconstruction: the scapular tip free flap. Head Neck. 2013;35(7):980–6. https://doi.org/10.1002/hed.23065.
8. Eskander A, Kang SY, Ozer E, et al. Supine positioning for the subscapular system of flaps: a pictorial essay. Head Neck. 2018;40(5):1068–72. https://doi.org/10.1002/hed.25051.
9. Feng AL, Nasser HB, Casper KA, et al. Lateral border and scapular tip free flaps: old school versus new school. Head Neck. 2022;44(2):576–81. https://doi.org/10.1002/hed.26905.
10. Stevens JR, Rosko AJ, Marchiano E, et al. The spider limb positioner in subscapular system free flaps. Oral Oncol. 2018;85:24–8. https://doi.org/10.1016/j.oraloncology.2018.08.004.
11. Rowsell AR, Davies DM, Eisenberg N, Taylor GI. The anatomy of the subscapular-thoracodorsal arterial system: study of 100 cadaver dissections. Br J Plast Surg. 1984;37(4):574–6. https://doi.org/10.1016/0007-1226(84)90152-8.

32 Serratus Anterior with Rib Free Flap

Ryan Judd, Hilary C. McCrary, and Nolan B. Seim

History

- First introduced in the literature by Takayanagi et al. in 1982 [1, 2].
- Initially used for soft tissue reconstruction only, but in recent decades expanded to use with scapular tip or rib.

Indications and Benefits

- Reconstruction of a variety of soft tissue +/– bone defect including coverage for laryngectomy or great vessel exposure, cutaneous, scalp, and skull base defects [3, 4].
- Useful in salvage cases or cases of peripheral vascular disease when a fibula or osteocutaneous radial forearm cannot be used or is unavailable.
- Thin, pliable flap with long pedicle.
- Can be utilized for immediate facial reanimation in cases of facial nerve sacrifice [5].
  - Long thoracic nerve anastamosed to remaining proximal facial nerve branches and/or masseteric nerve.
- Long pedicle that can be lengthened by extending to thoracodorsal and subscapular system (up to 12–13 cm).
- Minimal donor site morbidity that can be optimized with postoperative physical therapy.
- Option to harvest additional soft tissue and/or bone from the thoracodorsal system flap for larger defects [2, 6].

Anatomy

- The serratus anterior is a large fan-shaped muscle that originates on the upper eight to ten ribs and inserts on the costal surface of the medial border of the scapula (Fig. 32.1).
  - Composed of individual slips of muscle that each attach to a single rib.
  - The slips to the ninth and tenth ribs are variably present and often small.
  - Lower third of muscle involved in upward rotation and abduction of the scapula [7].
  - Upper/lateral portion of muscle is covered by latissimus dorsi.
- The serratus muscle has dual blood supply with the upper portion supplied by the lateral thoracic artery and lower portion supplied by serratus branch of thoracodorsal artery.

R. Judd · N. B. Seim (✉)
Department of Otolaryngology- Head and Neck Surgery, The Ohio State University, Columbus, OH, USA
e-mail: nolan.seim@osumc.edu

H. C. McCrary
Department of Otolaryngology- Head and Neck Surgery, University of Utah, Salt Lake City, UT, USA

R. Rezaee, A. Tamaki (eds.), *Local, Regional, and Free Flaps for Head and Neck Reconstruction*,
https://doi.org/10.1007/978-3-032-03211-9_32

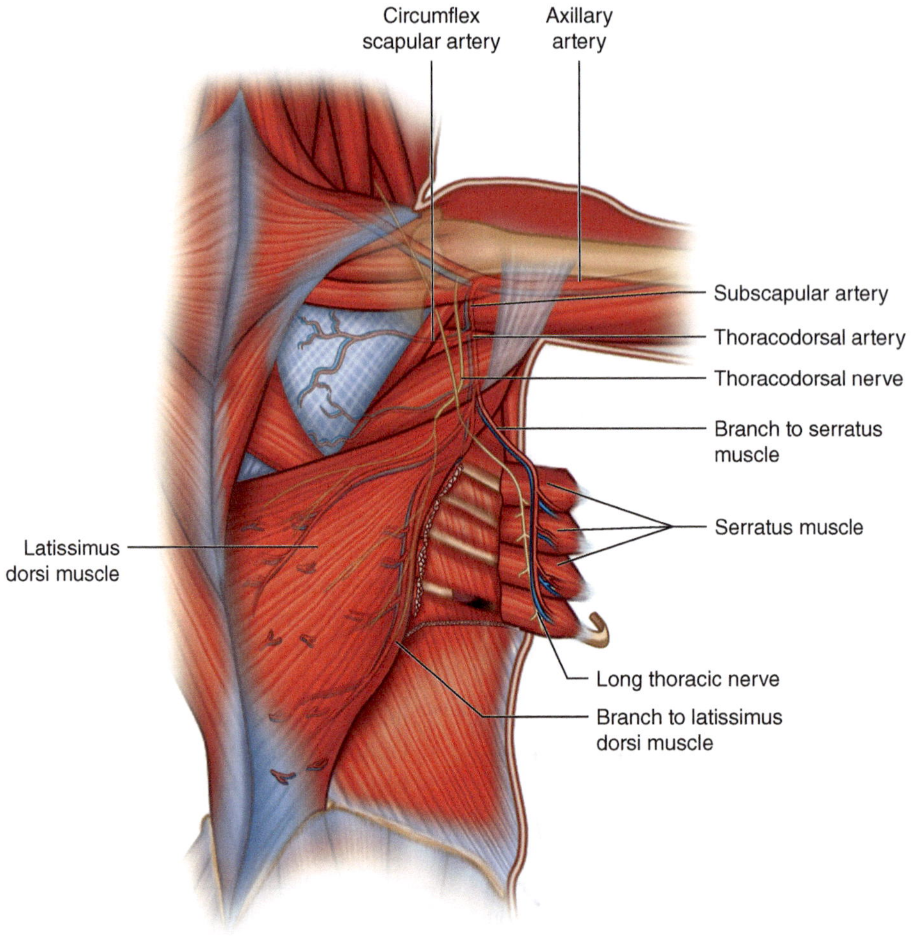

Fig. 32.1 The serratus anterior muscle is shown with the lower rib harvested. The sixth rib is most commonly harvested with the flap. Blood supply is via the branch to serratus muscle off of the thoracodorsal artery

  - Muscle slips originating from the fifth and sixth to the eighth, ninth, and tenth ribs are reliably supplied by the serratus branch of the thoracodorsal artery [1].
- Subscapular artery is a branch off the third part of the axillary artery.
  - Branches into circumflex scapular and thoracodorsal arteries.
  - Average length 2.2 cm before branching with a diameter of 3–4 mm.
  - Rarely, the thoracodorsal artery branches directly off the axillary artery (<5%) [8, 9].
- Thoracodorsal artery runs along the lateral surface of the scapula and deep surface of the latissimus dorsi, giving off several branches prior to entering the latissimus dorsi muscle at a neurovascular hilum [8].
  - Thoracodorsal vein enters lateral relative to the artery.
  - Thoracodorsal nerve is a branch of the posterior cord of the brachial plexus and runs with the vascular pedicle along the vein and artery.
- Serratus branch arises from the thoracodorsal artery.
  - Variability in number of branches: ~50% one branch, ~45% two branches, <5% three or more branches [8–10].
    - When there are multiple branches, there is typically a dominant branch that arborizes with the long thoracic nerve ("crow's foot" landmark) [9].

  - On average, arises 5.5 cm from the origin of the thoracodorsal artery.
  - 2 mm diameter at its origin from the thoracodorsal artery (1–3 mm range).
  - Mean pedicle length (from dominant serratus branch to circumflex scapular artery) is 11 cm.
  - Very rare reports of other vessels providing dominant blood supply to inferior serratus muscle slips [11].
- Serratus branch arteries are accompanied by paired venae comitantes, which unite to form a single thoracodorsal vein [8, 9].
- Long thoracic nerve is a branch of the brachial plexus (C5–C7).
  - Descends posterior to the axillary artery and vein.
  - Runs along anterior surface of serratus anterior, from medial to lateral as it descends.
  - Forms a "crow's foot" landmark where it intersects with the dominant serratus arterial branch [9].
    - Artery and nerve arborize simultaneously and resemble a crow's foot.
    - Nerve is most commonly deep to the vascular pedicle [9, 10].
- Ribs receive dual blood supply from the serratus branch and intercostal arteries via periosteal branches, which anastamose [12].

Preoperative Care

- Preoperative decision and protection of surgical arm (usually nondominant side however consider shape of rib bone if needed) to avoid placement of catheters.
- Assess for prior history of axillary dissection (e.g., breast cancer surgery or shoulder surgery).
- No need for specific testing preoperatively.
- Very low rates of atherosclerosis in the subscapular system.

Special Instruments and Positioning

- Can be harvested with supine positioning (+/− midline roll vs bean bag) to allow for two-surgeon approach. The ablative and reconstructive teams can then work concurrently for effective time management.
- Arm abducted and secured to arm board or arm holding device.

Modifications

- Can be harvested with bone (rib, scapular tip) [12, 14], nerve (long thoracic nerve) [13], latissimus dorsi muscle (for additional bulk) [15], or as part of a combination flap with the subscapular system [2, 6].

Pitfalls and Complications

- Rib can have poor bone perfusion.
  - The osteocutaneous serratus rib flap must be harvested with medial (anterior) rib as this is the location of the dense serratus muscle attachments and perforators to the bone.
  - The lateral (posterior) rib has only loose attachments to the muscle and few perforators and, therefore, should be limited in inclusion with the flap.
- The perforators to the skin can be small and variable in reliable perfusion. It is prudent to save the thoracodorsal pedicle to the latissimus dorsi myocutaneous flap until a skin paddle is successfully harvested with the serratus rib.
- Winged scapula can result from injury to the long thoracic nerve or over-resection of muscle.
  - Reduce risk by preserving upper slips of muscle to the scapula, which are not utilized in this flap.

  - Placing sutures between scapula and serratus is reported to promote fibrosis [3].
  - Postoperative physical therapy is helpful for optimal recovery.
- Risk of pneumothorax, particularly if rib harvested.
- Delayed identification of shoulder dysfunction can lead to worse functional outcomes. Higher risk of dysfunction with ipsilateral neck dissection. Any treatment-related shoulder dysfunction should be addressed with dedicated physical therapy [3, 16, 17].

Postoperative Care

- Closed suction drains with one drain often remaining in place at discharge.
- An abdominal binder can be used for several weeks to assist in reducing drain output and seating of the skin flaps.
- Prophylactic shoulder physical therapy for all patients.

Tissue type: *Myocutaneous, myofascial, osteocutaneous*
Artery: *Serratus anterior artery or thoracodorsal artery*
Vein: *Serratus anterior vein or thoracodorsal vein*
Nerve: *Long thoracic nerve*
Pedicle length: *Up to 12–13 cm (with dissection of the thoracodorsal artery and ligation of branches to the latissimus dorsi muscle and circumflex scapular artery up to the subscapular vascular system)*
Flap size: *Skin paddle size varies from patient to patient; however, skin paddles up to 20 × 20 cm have been reported*

Operative Procedure

1. The entire harvest of a serratus anterior flap can be completed in the supine position with the arm abducted on a padded arm board. The ablative and reconstructive teams can then work concurrently for effective time management.
2. When planning the incision, the anterior leading edge of the latissimus dorsi muscle should be palpated and marked. The incision traditionally courses along the anterior border of the latissimus dorsi muscle up into the axilla to assist with access to the thoracodorsal vascular pedicle.

   * However, if the patient has a higher body mass index, the incision can be made more anterior to account for the posterior skin flap hanging more posteriorly, improving access.

   * If harvesting a skin paddle, the skin paddle is traditionally harvested over the course of ribs 4–7. We recommend starting with only the posterior aspect of the incision until a perforator to the skin is identified. While a skin paddle has been described with this flap, this is unreliable and likely another flap option is a better choice if skin is needed for the reconstruction.

   * If planning for rib harvest, appropriate palpation and marking of ribs 5–8 should be completed, with the sixth rib being most commonly harvested with the flap.
3. Upon making incision, the first anatomical landmark is finding the anterior border of the latissimus dorsi muscle and retracting this posteriorly. The serratus anterior muscle will then be appreciated as it fans anteriorly, overlying the ribs (Fig. 32.1).
4. Identify the thoracodorsal artery and vein pedicle, with visualization of the branches going to the latissimus dorsi and serratus anterior muscle.

   * To increase pedicle length, the branches going to the latissimus dorsi muscle can be ligated, unless a chimeric flap is desired.
5. Once the pedicle and associated branching to the serratus anterior muscle are appreciated as well as the skin perforators, the anterior skin incision (if applicable) can be made.

   * Ensure the skin paddle does not sheer from the underlying perforators over ribs 4–7.
6. After assessing the volume of serratus anterior muscle necessary for harvest, dissect the muscle from the underlying ribs and posterior

scapular attachments from inferior to superior using electrocautery to ensure the vascular branches to the serratus anterior muscle are maintained. The long thoracic nerve will be encountered and may need to be ligated, especially for large flaps; however, it is recommended to preserve as much innervation as possible to the muscle not harvested. Prior authors have advocated that up to five muscle digitations can be harvested off a single vascular pedicle but size of flap should be based on visual distribution of the vascular pedicle as well [3].

Rib Harvest

(a) The muscular attachments to all the ribs, except for the rib planning to be harvested, are dissected. The periosteal blood supply arising from the serratus anterior muscle must be maintained.

* Most of the bone perforators are located medially (anteriorly) where the muscle is more densely attached to the rib.

(b) The length of the defect is confirmed, and this necessary length is marked out on the rib to be harvested. Create subperiosteal planes at the medial and lateral ends of the rib and place a malleable behind the rib to ensure there is no violation of the pleura.

(c) A saw is then used for osteotomies medially and laterally. The rib is carefully freed posteriorly from the pleural attachments.

* If a pleural defect occurs, can consider primary closure of the defect after air removed via drain vs chest tube. It is recommended to have a thoracic surgery consult intraoperatively if this situation occurs.

7. After the serratus anterior muscle is harvested and dissected free from underlying ribs (with or without rib harvest), the pedicle is dissected. Depending on the needs for the pedicle length, one can simply harvest the serratus anterior muscle branches arising from the thoracodorsal vessels or continue to trace it superiorly and harvest the pedicle from the thoracodorsal vessels just distal to the subscapular vasculature. The circumflex scapular vasculature can also be ligated as necessary to aid with pedicle length and size of vessel proximally.
8. Following harvest, place two suction drains in the wound. If a skin paddle is harvested, the anterior and posterior skin flaps can be undermined to allow for primary closure.

   * It is recommended to suture re-approximate the scapula to the chest wall to minimize the risk of winged scapula [2].

Disclosure Statement No conflicts of interest to disclose.

References

1. Takayanagi S, Tsukie T. Free serratus anterior muscle and myocutaneous flaps. Ann Plast Surg. 1982;8(4):277–83. https://doi.org/10.1097/00000637-198204000-00003.
2. Harii K, Ono I, Ebihara S. Closure of total cheek defects with two combined myocutaneous free flaps. Arch Otolaryngol. 1982;108(5):303–7. https://doi.org/10.1001/archotol.1982.00790530039010.
3. Khan MN, Rodriguez LG, Pool CD, et al. The versatility of the serratus anterior free flap in head and neck reconstruction. Laryngoscope. 2017;127(3):568–73. https://doi.org/10.1002/lary.26116.
4. Weber SM, Kim JH, Wax MK. Role of free tissue transfer in skull base reconstruction. Otolaryngol Head Neck Surg. 2007;136(6):914–9. https://doi.org/10.1016/j.otohns.2006.12.030.
5. Janik S, Marijic B, Faisal M, et al. Using the serratus anterior free flap for dynamic facial reanimation: systematic review. Head Neck. 2023;45(1):266–74. https://doi.org/10.1002/hed.27219.
6. Ilankovan V, Ramchandani P, Walji S, Anand R. Reconstruction of maxillary defects with serratus anterior muscle and angle of the scapula. Br J Oral Maxillofac Surg. 2011;49(1):53–7. https://doi.org/10.1016/j.bjoms.2009.10.034.
7. Ekstrom RA, Bifulco KM, Lopau CJ, Andersen CF, Gough JR. Comparing the function of the upper and lower parts of the serratus anterior muscle using surface electromyography. J Orthop Sports Phys Ther. 2004;34(5):235–43. https://doi.org/10.2519/jospt.2004.34.5.235.
8. Rowsell AR, Davies DM, Eisenberg N, Taylor GI. The anatomy of the subscapular-thoracodorsal arterial system: study of 100 cadaver dissections. Br J Plast Surg. 1984;37(4):574–6. https://doi.org/10.1016/0007-1226(84)90152-8.

9. Cuadros CL, Driscoll CL, Rothkopf DM. The anatomy of the lower serratus anterior muscle: a fresh cadaver study. Plast Reconstr Surg. 1995;95(1):93–7.
10. Erdogmus S, Govsa F. Distal variations of the neurovascular pedicle of the serratus anterior muscle as a flap. Surg Radiol Anat. 2005;27(2):100–7. https://doi.org/10.1007/s00276-004-0294-3.
11. Whitney TM, Buncke HJ, Alpert BS, Buncke GM, Lineaweaver WC. The serratus anterior free-muscle flap: experience with 100 consecutive cases. Plast Reconstr Surg. 1990;86(3):481–90.
12. Richards MA, Poole MD, Godfrey AM. The serratus anterior/rib composite flap in mandibular reconstruction. Br J Plast Surg. 1985;38(4):466–77. https://doi.org/10.1016/0007-1226(85)90002-5.
13. Janik SJ, Paraszti I, Hirtler L, et al. Design of skin islands for a myocutaneous serratus anterior free flap-an anatomical study and clinical implication for pharyngeal reconstruction after laryngopharyngectomy. Clin Otolaryngol. 2019;44(3):227–34. https://doi.org/10.1111/coa.13257.
14. Penfold CN, Davies HT, Cole RP, Evans BT, Hobby JA. Combined latissimus dorsi-serratus anterior/rib composite free flap in mandibular reconstruction. Int J Oral Maxillofac Surg. 1992;21(2):92–6. https://doi.org/10.1016/s0901-5027(05)80540-5.
15. Kim PD, Blackwell KE. Latissimus-serratus-rib free flap for oromandibular and maxillary reconstruction. Arch Otolaryngol Head Neck Surg. 2007;133(8):791–5. https://doi.org/10.1001/archotol.133.8.791.
16. Derby LD, Bartlett SP, Low DW. Serratus anterior free-tissue transfer: harvest-related morbidity in 34 consecutive cases and a review of the literature. J Reconstr Microsurg. 1997;13(6):397–403. https://doi.org/10.1055/s-2007-1006419.
17. Dumont CE, Domenghini C, Kessler J. Donor site morbidity after serratus anterior free muscular flap: a prospective clinical study. Ann Plast Surg. 2004;52(2):195–8. https://doi.org/10.1097/01.sap.0000096378.59694.54.

33 Temporal Artery Posterior Auricular Skin Free Flap

Jamil Hayden and Shawn Li

History

- A pedicled retroauricular skin flap based on the superficial temporal artery was first described in 1969 by Washio [1]. This was a rotational flap that required a two-staged approach and was primarily used for nasal reconstruction.
- The temporal artery posterior auricular skin (TAPAS) flap was first introduced in the literature by Lassus et al. in 2016 [2].

Indications and Benefits

- Reconstruction of small- to medium-sized intraoral and facial defects.
- Thin, well vascularized, and pliable tissue.
- Benefits of non-hair bearing tissue with good skin color match for facial defects. For intraoral defects, good pliability and beneficial lack of bulk.
- Potential for restoring the gingivobuccal sulcus in secondary oral cavity reconstruction.
- Consistent and reliable vascular anatomy.
  - The average reported pedicle length was 6 cm, with a mean diameter of 1.8 mm for the artery and 2.2 mm for the vein [3].
  - The maximum safe skin paddle size was 4 × 7 cm with an average thickness of 3 mm [4].
- Limited donor site morbidity.

Anatomy

- The TAPAS flap is composed of postauricular skin and is supplied by the superior auricular artery and its vascular anastomoses with the posterior auricular artery (Fig. 33.1).
- The skin paddle is centered over the retroauricular sulcus. The skin paddle borders:
  - Anteriorly to the posterior aspect of the pinna 5 mm behind and parallel to the auricular rim
  - Posteriorly to the postauricular skin or up to the hairline
  - Superiorly to the helical attachment to the temporal skin
  - Inferiorly to where the concha ends at the mastoid process

J. Hayden
Ear, Nose and Throat Institute, University Hospitals Cleveland Medical Center, Cleveland, OH, USA

Case Western Reserve University School of Medicine, Cleveland, OH, USA

Department of Otolaryngology-HNS, Penn State Health, Hershey, PA, USA

S. Li (✉)
Department of Otolaryngology- Head and Neck Surgery, Penn State Health, Hershey, PA, USA
e-mail: Shawnli@pennstatehealth.psu.edu

R. Rezaee, A. Tamaki (eds.), *Local, Regional, and Free Flaps for Head and Neck Reconstruction*,
https://doi.org/10.1007/978-3-032-03211-9_33

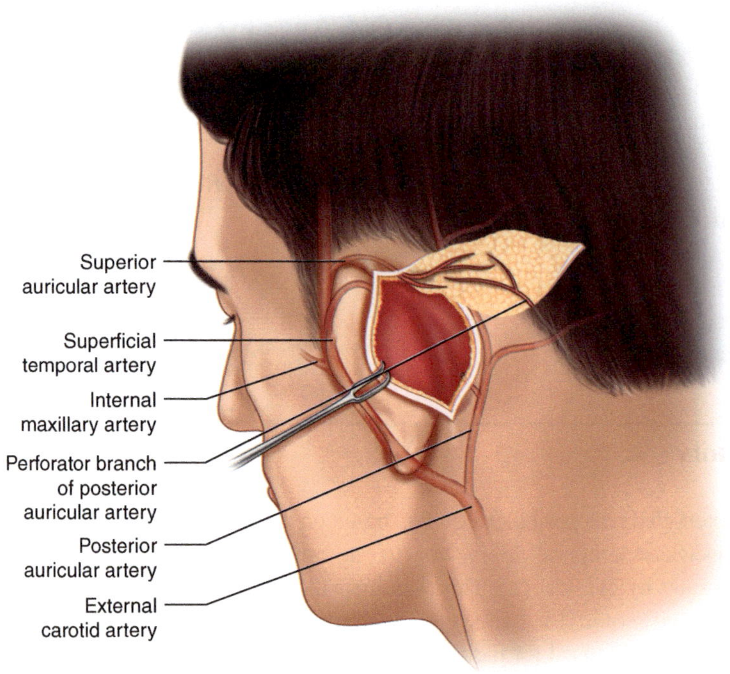

Fig. 33.1 Elevation of the TAPAS flap based off the superficial temporal blood supply

- The superficial temporal artery and the posterior auricular artery are branches of the external carotid artery.
- The blood supply of the auricle consists of branches from the superficial temporal artery as well as the posterior auricular artery.
  - The superficial temporal artery gives off three branches that supply the anterior surface of the auricle: the superior auricular artery, middle auricular artery, and inferior auricular artery.
  - The superior auricular artery is a branch off the superficial temporal artery that was first described in 1996 by Song et al. [5].
  - There are reported cases of anatomic variations in the arterial supply including reverse pedicle blood flow and the pedicle arising from the frontal or parietal branches of the superficial temporal artery [6].
- The venous drainage of the TAPAS flap is typically from the superficial temporal vein, but in a few cases, the posterior auricular vein has been noted to be the main source of drainage and can serve as a second vein for anastomosis.
  - There are also reported anomalies with the superficial temporal vein, where the vein has been absent or reported to be up to 3 cm posterior to the superficial temporal artery [7].
- Sensory innervation is derived from the auriculotemporal nerve.
  - The auriculotemporal nerve can be incorporated to produce a sensate TAPAS flap, yet this should only be used in cases where sacrifice of the distal auriculotemporal nerve is required for flap harvest.

Preoperative Care

- Assess for history or scars from prior surgery or trauma that may compromise vascular anatomy or perfusion to the skin.

Special Instruments and Positioning

- The entire ear is prepped into the surgical field. A portion of the hair around the surgical field may need to be shaved.

Modifications

- Can harvest conchal cartilage for a composite flap. This can be particularly useful in nasal reconstruction.

Pitfalls and Complications

- Potential for anatomical variation of the vasculature.
- Initial transient venous stasis has been reported [2].
- Given the thinness of the flap, the skin has a blue hue that can make postoperative monitoring difficult.
- The length of the pedicle is short, so it is only suitable for small- to medium-sized defects.

Postoperative Care

- If a skin graft is used over the postauricular donor site, apply a bolster.
  - Dressing and bolster are generally removed within 5 to 7 days, but some may continue for longer.
- If a closed suction drain is used, it should be removed after 1 to 3 days based on output.

Tissue type: *Fasciocutaneous*
Artery: *Superior auricular artery, posterior auricular artery*
Vein: *Superficial temporal vein, posterior auricular vein*
Nerve: *Auriculotemporal nerve*
Pedicle length: *5.5 to 6 cm*
Flap size: *Maximum reported 4 × 7 cm*

Operative Procedure

1. Plan a skin flap centered on the retroauricular sulcus. The anterior portion of the skin flap extends over the retroauricular skin up to 5 mm posterior to the helical rim. The posterior extent of the skin flap includes the postauricular skin and can extend to the postauricular hairline. Flap measurements are adjusted based on the size of the surgical defect.
2. A preauricular incision is marked from the auriculocephalic groove down to the attachment of the lobule. This preauricular incision may extend superiorly and anteriorly across the hairline to allow for better exposure of the superficial temporal vessels.
3. The preauricular skin incision is made. The superficial temporal vessels are visualized and dissected proximally to the maxillary branches. The dissection then continues distally, in a cranial direction. Small branches supplying the tragus are ligated (Fig. 33.1).

   * Care is taken to preserve the subcutaneous tissue near the helical root to avoid injury to vasculature supplying the flap.
4. The postauricular skin incision is made. An anterior curvilinear incision is made on the retroauricular skin and a posterior curvilinear incision is made on the postauricular skin and the incisions are connected inferiorly. Starting from the inferior aspect of the flap, the depth of the flap is established not to violate the post-auricular muscular attachments at the mastoid tip. The flap is then elevated in a retrograde fashion from inferior to superior.

   * Care is taken to limit the amount of cautery used to preserve the vasculature to the thin flap.

   * Perichondrium is left behind on the auricular cartilage.

   * Minor branches of the helical arcade will be encountered and clipped as the flap is elevated superiorly.
5. The skin of the helical root is then incorporated into the superior aspect of the flap by

elevating this skin in a sub-perichondrial plane. The anterior skin incision is brought down to the auricular cartilage.

* While the postauricular elevation is supra-perichondrial, it must transition to sub-perichondrial at the helix to minimize the chance for pedicle/perforator damage at this location.

6. The dissection is then continued anteriorly, superficial to the temporalis fascia. Distal branches of the superficial temporal artery encountered during this portion of the dissection are clipped and divided.
7. Preauricular fascial attachments are released, and the proximal end of the superficial temporal artery is dissected down and separated from the superficial temporal vein. Care is taken to avoid injury to the facial nerve.
8. At this point, the postauricular portion of the flap should be completely mobilized and separated, while its vascular pedicle remains intact until decision for rotation or free flap is made.

   * The flap may be used as a rotational or free flap based on the location and size of the defect.

   * For central defects, the angular artery and regional veins or distal facial system can be suitable for anastomoses.
9. Following harvest, the postauricular donor site is then closed primarily. Alternatively, a split thickness skin graft (0.12–0.20 inch thickness) can be used if primary closure is not feasible. Additionally, a small suction drain can be placed. The preauricular incision is closed primarily.

Disclosure Statement No conflicts of interest to disclose.

References

1. Washio H. Retroauricular-temporal flap. Plast Reconstr Surg. 1969;43(2):162–6. https://doi.org/10.1097/00006534-196902000-00009.
2. Lassus P, Lindford AJ. Free temporal artery posterior auricular skin (TAPAS) flap: a new option in facial and intra-oral reconstruction. Microsurgery. 2017;37(6):525–30. https://doi.org/10.1002/micr.30069.
3. Lassus P, Husso A, Vuola J, Lindford AJ. More than just the helix: a series of free flaps from the ear. Microsurgery. 2018;38(6):611–20. https://doi.org/10.1002/micr.30178.
4. Ganry L, Ettinger KS, Rougier G, Qassemyar Q, Fernandes RP. Revisiting the temporal artery posterior auricular skin flap with an anatomical basis stepwise pedicle dissection for use in targeted facial subunit reconstruction. Head Neck. 2020;42(11):3153–60. https://doi.org/10.1002/hed.26362.
5. Song R, Song Y, Qi K, Jiang H, Pan F. The superior auricular artery and retroauricular arterial Island flaps. Plast Reconstr Surg. 1996;98(4):657–67; discussion 668–70. https://doi.org/10.1097/00006534-199609001-00009.
6. Kilinc H, Bilen BT. A new approach to retroauricular flap transfer: parietal branch-based reverse flow superior auricular artery Island flap. Ann Plast Surg. 2006;56(4):380–3. https://doi.org/10.1097/01.sap.0000202147.15402.50.
7. Boeckx W. Temporoparietal artery perforator flap. In: Perforator flaps: anatomy, technique and clinical applications, vol. I. Quality Medical Publishing, Inc; 2006. p. 200–15.

Thoracodorsal Artery Perforator Free Flap

34

Eric M. Dowling and Jonathan C. Garneau

History

- The thoracodorsal artery perforator (TDAP) flap was first described in the literature by Angrigiani et al. and Spinelli in 1995 [1, 2].
- The harvest of this flap was initially described as a latissimus dorsi myocutaneous flap without muscle. As perforator flaps emerged within reconstructive surgery, the flap was described as a muscle-sparing harvest technique to obtain fasciocutaneous or myocutaneous (with limited muscle) flaps in the latissimus dorsi (LD) anatomic region.

Indications and Benefits

- Depending on a patient's body habitus, the TDAP fasciocutaneous skin paddle may be of intermediate thickness with excellent pliability.
  - The thickness is greater than that of a radial forearm and typically less than that of an anterolateral thigh donor site.
  - The tissue quality is similar to that of a lateral arm flap.
- Pedicle length and vessel caliber is excellent for nearly all head and neck defects.
- The clear advantages of the donor site are as follows:
  - The majority of donor sites can be closed primarily.
  - The perforator dissection is muscle-sparing and nerve-sparing. This preserves LD muscle function and limits morbidity.
  - The surgical scar is hidden in a cosmetically favorable location in the scapular region.
- The TDAP flap can be harvested as a single fasciocutaneous flap or part of a chimeric flap from the thoracodorsal vascular system. This skin paddle is an excellent option in conjunction with the scapular tip flap if osteocutaneous reconstruction is required. Since the skin paddle is supplied through the thoracodorsal system, a chimeric scapular tip flap can be harvested without supply of the circumflex scapular system.

Anatomy

- The thoracodorsal artery arises from the subscapular artery, which is the largest branch of the axillary artery.
  - However, in 0.8–3% of cases, the thoracodorsal artery may arise directly from the axillary artery [3].

E. M. Dowling · J. C. Garneau (✉)
Department of Otolaryngology- Head and Neck Surgery, University of Virginia Health System, Charlottesville, VA, USA
e-mail: jcg6j@uvahealth.org

R. Rezaee, A. Tamaki (eds.), *Local, Regional, and Free Flaps for Head and Neck Reconstruction*,
https://doi.org/10.1007/978-3-032-03211-9_34

- The thoracodorsal artery will enter the LD muscle and divide into transverse and vertical (descending) branches in most cases. This division within the muscle can form the basis for two separate myocutaneous or fasciocutaneous perforator flaps from the same system (Fig. 34.1).
  - The perforators arising from the vertical (descending) LD branch of the thoracodorsal tend to have a shorter intramuscular course than the transverse branch, thus are favorable for intramuscular perforator dissection.
- Mean pedicle length is estimated at 15 cm (this assumes maximal dissection to the axillary artery origin).
- Perforators are localized based on the following:
  - Perforators are located 8–10 cm below the axillary fold.
  - 4 cm inferior to the scapular tip and 1–2 cm from the anterior leading edge of the LD muscle [4].
  - The highest density of perforators (>0.5 mm in diameter) are typically located 9.5–15.4 cm from the posterior axillary fold within 4.3 cm of the anterior border of the LD muscle [5].
  - Septocutaneous perforators may exist in the avascular plane between the LD and serratus anterior (SA) muscle. Therefore, care should be taken to evaluate this region

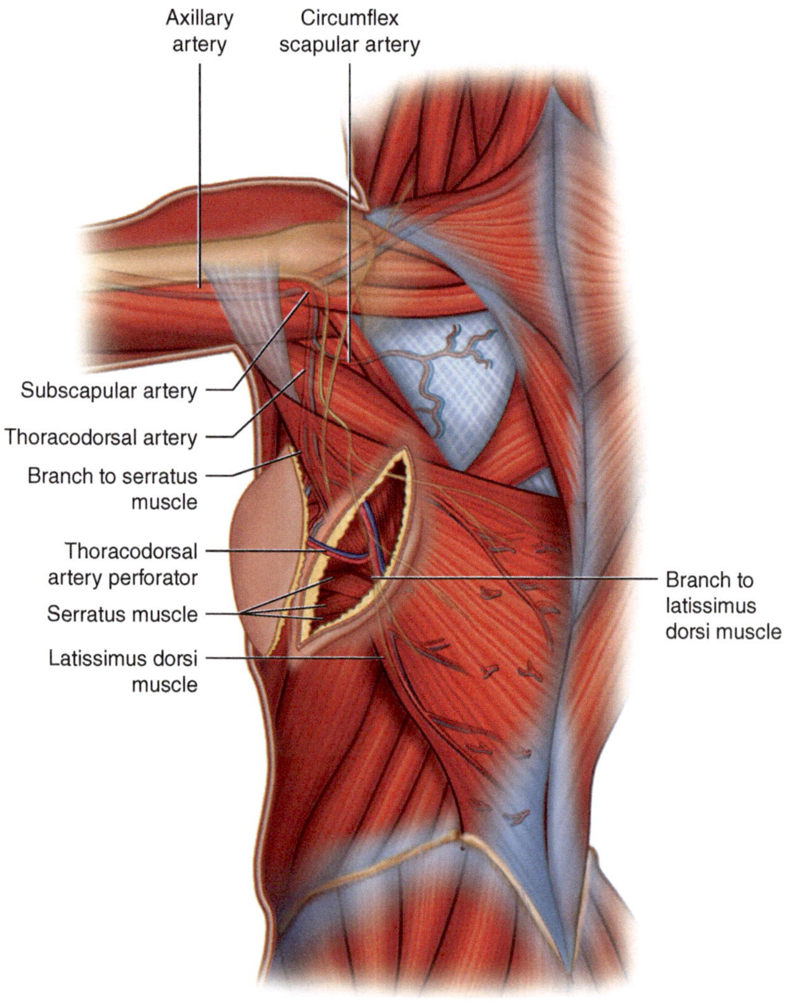

Fig. 34.1 The fasciocutaneous thoracodorsal artery perforator flap is demonstrated here and isolated on its vascular pedicle. The perforator has been dissected through the latissimus dorsi muscle and freed from surrounding tissue to demonstrate its origin from the latissimus dorsi branch of thoracodorsal artery/vein

while defining the anterior leading edge of the LD and prior to dissecting over the LD muscle to identify the (more common) musculocutaneous perforators.
  - If a robust septocutaneous perforator is found, this considerably simplifies the dissection and harvest of this flap as the traditional intramuscular perforator dissection is not required.

Preoperative Care

- No preoperative imaging is required.
- Physical examination of the region is recommended to evaluate for any prior surgical incisions, skin thickness, quality for the anticipated defect, and preoperative limitations of shoulder mobility or upper extremity range of motion.
- Determine whether the patient is right- or left-hand dominant. Most prefer to harvest from the nondominant side unless circumstances dictate otherwise. For instance, prior surgery (or flap harvest), preoperative range of motion difficulties, or intraoperative patient positioning may factor into this decision.

Special Instruments and Positioning

- The dominant perforator(s) can be identified with a handheld Doppler probe prior to flap design and incisions.
- Simultaneous harvest of the TDAP flap can be performed with a second team during the ablative procedure with thoughtful positioning and team communication.
- An intraoperative assistant, Mayo stand, or limb holder apparatus can be used to assist with arm positioning intraoperatively and limit the need for lateral decubitus positioning [2, 6].
- Traditionally, the most described harvest position is the lateral decubitus position. This can be facilitated by placing an inflatable bean bag on the bed prior to patient positioning. Additional hip bump placement can enhance rotation. An axillary roll is typically placed to avoid compression of the contralateral upper extremity during the harvest.

Modifications

- TDAP can be one of several components within a chimeric scapular-based flap.
- TDAP flap can be incorporated into the osteocutaneous scapular tip flap if osteocutaneous reconstruction is needed. There is more freedom and separation of the skin paddle from the osseous component, allowing for more complex flap designs.
- Multiple perforators can be identified to allow for separate skin paddles for larger or more complex, multi-paddle reconstructions.
- The underlying LD muscle can be incorporated into the flap, but with knowledge of the perforator, the skin paddle can be partially separated from the underlying muscle, allowing for more rotation or freedom of the fasciocutaneous component from the underlying muscle.

Pitfalls and Complications

- Fragile or diminutive perforator supply to the skin paddle that may be susceptible to injury.
- Need for tedious intramuscular dissection of the perforator.
- Risk of kinking, twisting, or compression of the perforator once inset into the head and neck defect.
- Partial loss of the flap at potential watershed areas based on perforator supply.
  - If available, infrared perfusion technology can be used if perfusion is in question including in larger flaps.
- Suboptimal patient positioning, making harvest labor intensive or ergonomically unfavorable.

Postoperative Care

- Drain placement within the donor site is required.
- Primary closure can be achieved in nearly all cases with development of bilateral advancement flaps. Inferior and superior extended back cuts can be made to facilitate closure.
  - If a skin graft is required, placement of a wound vacuum device is recommended to stabilize the graft and avoid excessive motion along the skin graft that can result from upper extremity movements.
- Although not required, an upper extremity "arm immobilizer" can be employed if there is concern that excessive motion may place stress along the closure. However, in the majority of cases, very limited postoperative care of the donor site is required.

Tissue type: *Adipofascial, fasciocutaneous, myocutaneous*
Artery: *Thoracodorsal artery*
Vein: *Thoracodorsal vein*
Nerve: *Thoracodorsal nerve*
Pedicle length: *15 cm (if dissected to the axillary artery)*
Flap size: *Upward of 15 × 25 cm*

Operative Procedure

1. External landmarks are palpated and marked (anterior border of the LD muscle, axilla, posterior axillary fold, scapular tip). The flap can be oriented vertically (cranio-caudally) or horizontally (antero-posteriorly) depending on the defect and complexity of the skin paddle design.

   * Once flap design and measurements are made, handheld Doppler can be used to confirm the perforator(s) are properly captured with the flap design [7].
2. Incision is made along the anterior border of the LD muscle. The incision should be made broadly to provide wide exposure during initial flap elevation. The incision should be through the skin and subcutaneous fat, keeping in mind that septocutaneous TDAP perforators may be present between the septum of the SA and LD muscle.
3. The plane between the SA and LD is identified. The anterior border of the LD muscle is defined and followed along the anterior border along the LD fascia. The LD muscle is retracted anteriorly (ventrally), while the skin flap is raised in the anterior to posterior direction. This should be done under loupe magnification, with caution while dissecting along the anterior border and anticipating a dominant musculocutaneous perforator 1–2 cm inside the LD muscle.
4. If a robust perforator is observed, it can be dissected through the LD muscle toward its origin. Meticulous dissection along the perforator through the muscle is performed, while intervening muscle fibers are divided with fine bipolar cautery. The perforator is traced to its origin of the LD branch of the thoracodorsal vascular pedicle (typically the vertical branch). Once the origin of the perforator is defined and mapped to its origin on the surface of the LD muscle, the adjacent branches of the thoracodorsal artery/vein can be ligated so that the perforator is isolated on its main blood supply (Fig. 34.1).

   * A small portion of the muscle can be left adjacent to the dissected intramuscular component of the perforator based on surgeon preference and comfort.
5. The thoracodorsal artery and vein are then traced along its path from the LD muscle to the axilla. Along the dissection, the angular vessels, SA vessels, and smaller contributions to teres muscle will be encountered and will need to be isolated, ligated, and divided.
6. The perforator can be released from its surrounding LD muscle. This can be done while ligating small perforating branches to the LD muscle, or a small cuff of muscle can be left along the pedicle as a layer of protection and perforator stabilization.
7. The dissection of the thoracodorsal artery and vein can be guided by the thoracodorsal nerve to the LD. The nerve can be easily found and traced to the axilla.

Identification and dissection along the nerve can proceed rapidly and provide safe protection of the vascular pedicle. The nerve is typically spared in this flap harvest, once the path is dissected, the nerve can be carefully freed from the pedicle and preserved.

8. The majority of the flap has been raised, thus far, without committing to the final dimensions of the flap based on the defect. Once the perforator is fully defined and the defect is known, the posterior cut on the skin paddle can be made. The perforator is captured and the skin paddle is elevated from the underlying LD muscle posteriorly. The flap can be elevated from posterior to anterior and fully isolated on its vascular pedicle.
9. The proximal dissection of the pedicle will proceed to the axillary artery. If a long pedicle is not needed, vessels can be dissected to the level of the subscapular artery/vein and vessels are ligated distal to the circumflex scapular artery. If larger caliber vessel diameter or increased pedicle length is needed, the subscapular vessels can be further dissected.

   * The circumflex scapular artery can be dissected and even add additional arterial pedicle length and/or provide more favorable vessel size match via a retrograde arterial anastomosis.
10. The flap is harvested and the back can be closed primarily in the majority of cases.

Disclosure Statement No conflicts of interest to disclose.

References

1. Angrigiani C, Grilli D, Siebert J. Latissimus dorsi musculocutaneous flap without muscle. Plast Reconstr Surg. 1995;96:1608–11.
2. Spinelli HM, Fink JA, Muzaffar AR. The latissimus dorsi perforator- based fasciocutaneous flap. Ann Plast Surg. 1996;37:500~.
3. O'Connel JE, Bajwa MS, Schache AG, Shaw RJ. Head and neck reconstruction with free flaps based on the thoracodorsal system. Oral Oncol. 2017;75:46–53.
4. Heitmann C, Guerra A, Metzinger SW, Levin LS, Allen RJ. The thoracodorsal artery perforator flap: anatomic basis and clinical application. Ann Plast Surg. 2003;51(1):23–9.
5. Schaverien M, Wong C, Bailey S, Saint-Cyr M. Thoracodorsal artery perforator flap and latissimus dorsi myocutaneous flap – anatomical study of the constant skin paddle perforator locations. J Plast Reconstr Aesthet Surg. 2010;63(12):2123–7.
6. Stevens JR, Rosko AJ, Marchiano E, Haring C, Chinn SB, Mallow KM, Prince ME, Casper K, Moyer J, Chepeha D, Stucken CL, Spector ME. The spider limb positioner in subscapular system free flaps. Oral Oncol. 2018;85:24–8.
7. Guyonvarch P, Kolb F. Thoracodorsal artery perforator free flap with vascularized thoracodorsal nerve for head and neck reconstruction following radical parotidectomy with facial nerve sacrifice: step by step surgical technique video. Head Neck. 2021;43(7):2255–8.

Ulnar Forearm Free Flap 35

Emily J. Marchiano and Brittany Barber

History

- The ulnar fasciocutaneous free flap was first described by Lovie et al. in 1984 as an alternative to the mainstay radial forearm free flap (RFFF) [1].

Indications and Benefits

- Reconstruction application is identical to the RFFF and includes both mucosal (oral cavity, oropharynx, larynx, pharynx, skull base) and cutaneous defects.
- Nearly indistinguishable tissue characteristics from the RFFF—thin and pliable soft tissue with wide application for use.
- Predictable vascular anatomy.
  - Long pedicle measuring 10–12 cm in length (approximately 4 cm shorter than the RFFF) and large caliber arterial pedicle with approximately 2.5 mm diameter [2]. The vein caliber is variable and typically the larger of the two venae comitantes (1–2 mm) is utilized for microvascular anastomosis. The mean number of perforators is 4.3 [3].
- Superior morbidity outcomes have been reported in the ulnar forearm free flap (UFFF) compared to the RFFF, including improved cosmesis, less risk of tendon exposure, and less hair density of harvested skin paddle [6].
- Possibility for multiple skin paddles based off single vascular pedicle [4].

Anatomy

- The brachial artery, a continuation of the axillary artery, branches into the radial and ulnar artery approximately 2–3 cm below the elbow (Fig. 35.1).
- The ulnar artery originates at the level of the radial neck and is accompanied by two venae comitantes.
- In the proximal forearm, the vascular pedicle is deep to the pronator teres, flexor carpi radialis, and flexor digitorum superficialis. Distally, it travels superficial to the flexor digitorum profundus muscle belly and can be identified between the flexor carpi ulnaris and the flexor digitorum superficialis [7].
- The ulnar artery septocutaneous perforators can be found along a line from the pisiform bone to the medial epicondyle, approximately 7–15 cm proximal to the pisiform [4].
- The flap is thought to primarily drain from the deep system. The artery is accompanied by paired venae comitantes. These do not always

E. J. Marchiano · B. Barber (✉)
Department of Otolaryngology- Head and Neck Surgery, University of Washington, Seattle, WA, USA
e-mail: bbarber1@uw.edu

R. Rezaee, A. Tamaki (eds.), *Local, Regional, and Free Flaps for Head and Neck Reconstruction*,
https://doi.org/10.1007/978-3-032-03211-9_35

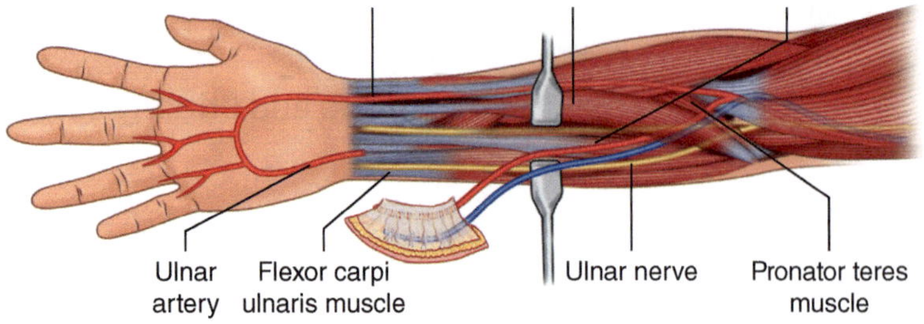

Fig. 35.1 Ulnar fasciocutaneous free flap harvest demonstrating close association of the vascular pedicle to the unlar nerve housed between the flexor carpi ulnaris and flexor digitorum superficialis muscles

converge and anastomosis may need to be performed utilizing the larger of the two venae.
  - The basilic vein is a large superficial vein draining the ulnar forearm region. The course of the basilic vein is typically inconsistent and therefore, most rely primarily on the deep system for venous drainage of the flap [4, 5]. However, if present in adequate length and caliber, the basilic vein can be harvested with the UFFF and a second anastomosis can be performed.
- The ulnar nerve enters the forearm posterior to the medial epicondyle.
  - It is a mixed sensory and motor nerve. It innervates the flexor carpi ulnaris, ulnar half of the flexor digitorum, interossei, adductor pollicis, and ulnar-sided lumbrical muscles. It provides sensory innervation to the fifth digit and the ulnar half of the ring finger and ulnar half of the hand.
  - The ulnar nerve joins the ulnar artery in the proximal forearm and accompanies it along its entire course in the forearm.
  - The dorsal branch of the ulnar nerve (DBUN; sensory innervation to the dorsum of the hand) arises from the ulnar nerve, 8–9 cm from the pisiform bone. The DBUN divides into two dorsal digital branches, one of which provides the cutaneous innervation of the dorsum of the fifth digit, and the other, the cutaneous innervation of the medial half of the fourth digit. An anatomic variant exists wherein the DBUN travels around the ulnar proximal to the ulnar styloid process [5].
- Sensory innervation of the flap is supplied by the medial cutaneous nerve of the forearm, which runs with the basilic vein.
- The ulnar artery terminates in the superficial palmar arch, while the radial artery terminates in the deep palmar arch. Communication between these systems is essential for maintaining vascularity of the hand following sacrifice of either artery.
- Anatomic variation:
  - Superficial ulnar artery is an anatomic variant encountered in 0.7–9.0% of cases and is of relevance because inadvertent injury can occur easily during flap harvest [8].
  - Martin-Gruber anastomosis (MGA; anastomosis between ulnar and radial nerves located in the proximal third of the forearm) observed in 11.5–27% of cases [5, 9]. The connecting branches of the MGA run deep to the vascular pedicle of the UFFF and can always be preserved.

Preoperative Care

- An Allen's test should be performed to understand the ability of the hand to be perfused by either the ulnar or radial artery.
  - In performing this test, the arm should be lifted above the heart while occluding both vessels, release of the radial artery should result in reperfusion of the hand within 15 s. This should be performed again, except with release of the ulnar artery instead.

  - If there is doubt about the results of an Allen's test, a preoperative vascular ultrasound can be utilized.
- Patient history including handedness, prior surgery, and trauma are important to decision-making about which arm to utilize and protection of the surgical arm preoperatively.
  - An arm band can be used to prevent IV and blood draws from the operative hand.
  - The nondominant hand is typically utilized.
- The hair density is less with a more proximally located skin paddle.

Special Instruments and Positioning

- Utilization of a tourniquet (250 mmHg, limit <2 h) is surgeon preference. Esmarch wrap or ace wrap can be used to exsanguinate the arm prior to inflation of the tourniquet.
- Supine positioning allows the arm to be prepped on an arm board. This is extended out during harvest.

Modifications

- This can be harvested as a sensate flap (medial cutaneous nerve of the forearm), with tendon (palmaris longus) or muscle (flexor carpi ulnaris). Although described in conjunction with vascularized bone, the ulnar bone stock is even less than the radius and is not routinely performed [2].
- A split thickness skin graft can be elevated from the flap such that only the deep fascia and subcutaneous tissue is harvested.
- Separate skin paddles can be utilized for monitoring the flap or for reconstruction of fistulous defects when used for pharyngo-esophageal reconstruction [10, 11].

Pitfalls and Complications

- Ischemic hand.
- Hypoesthesia of the hand.
- Tendon exposure and wound healing complications. Depending on the size of the defect, the UFFF can be harvested such that exposure of the tendon of the flexor carpi ulnaris is limited decreasing the risk of this complication.
- Decreased grip strength. Although this has been shown to normalize after 6 months in all fingers [12].

Postoperative Care

- A bolster or negative pressure wound therapy can be placed on the forearm skin. These are removed after 5 days.
- A volar splint or cast is placed over the forearm holding the wrist in slight extension.
- A proximally located suction drain is placed and removed within 5 days.

Tissue type: *Adipofascial, fasciocutaneous*
Artery: *Ulnar artery*
Vein: *Venae comitantes, basilic vein*
Nerve: *Medial nerve to the forearm*
Pedicle length: *10–14 cm*
Flap size: *Skin paddle from antecubital fossa to flexor crease. Maximum reported 9 × 22 cm*

Operative Procedure

1. A line drawn from the pisiform at the wrist to the medial epicondyle describes the most common location of the perforators. A skin paddle centered on this line is planned based on surgeon preference. Proximally, a curvilinear incision is made toward the antecubital fossa.

   * The UFFF has a shorter pedicle compared to the RFFF and the incision often does not need to be extended all the way to the antecubital fossa.
2. The skin incision is made on the radial aspect of the flap, and the incision is carried down to the muscle belly of the flexor digitorum superficialis.
3. The dissection proceeds from the radial to ulnar direction suprafascially until the perforators and ulnar artery are identified.
4. Once identified, the ulnar aspect of the incision can be made and carried down to the flexor carpi ulnaris.

5. The vascular pedicle can be identified between the flexor carpi ulnaris (ulnarly) and flexor digitorum superficialis (radially).
   * The artery is housed in a thin fascial septum.
   * It is essential at this point to take care not to injury the fasciocutaneous perforators that arise from the vascular pedicle.
6. The ulnar nerve will be seen immediately adjacent to the artery.
7. The vascular pedicle is ligated and divided distally.
   * If performed without a tourniquet, an intraoperative Allen's test can be performed prior to ligation.
8. The dissection proceeds distal to proximal and the vascular pedicle is carefully dissected from the ulnar nerve. Particular care is taken in this portion of the dissection and small vessels to the nerve are clipped.
9. The dissection continues until the common interosseous artery is identified.
   * If on tourniquet, this can be released to reperfuse the flap and the distal hand is evaluated for adequate blood flow.
10. The flap is harvested at the bifurcation between the ulnar artery and the common interosseous artery.
11. The proximal donor site is closed primarily and the defect is closed either primarily or with a skin graft (either full or split thickness grafts are described).

Disclosure Statement No conflicts of interest to disclose.

References

1. Lovie MJ, Duncan GM, Glasson DW. The ulnar artery forearm free flap. Br J Plast Surg. 1984;37(4):486–92. https://doi.org/10.1016/0007-1226(84)90136-x.
2. Sieg P, Bierwolf S. Ulnar versus radial forearm flap in head and neck reconstruction: an experimental and clinical study. Head Neck. 2001;23(11):967–71. https://doi.org/10.1002/hed.1140.
3. Huang JJ, Wu CW, Lam WL, et al. Anatomical basis and clinical application of the ulnar forearm free flap for head and neck reconstruction. Laryngoscope. 2012;122(12):2670–6. https://doi.org/10.1002/lary.23565.
4. Yu P, Chang EI, Selber JC, Hanasono MM. Perforator patterns of the ulnar artery perforator flap. Plast Reconstr Surg. 2012;129(1):213–20. https://doi.org/10.1097/PRS.0b013e3182362a9c.
5. Hakim SG, Trenkle T, Sieg P, Jacobsen HC. Ulnar artery-based free forearm flap: review of specific anatomic features in 322 cases and related literature. Head Neck. 2014;36(8):1224–9. https://doi.org/10.1002/hed.23594.
6. Xu Q, Chen PL, Liu YH, Wang SM, Xu ZF, Feng CJ. Comparing donor site morbidity between radial and ulnar forearm free flaps: a meta-analysis. Br J Oral Maxillofac Surg. 2022;60(5):547–53. https://doi.org/10.1016/j.bjoms.2021.10.014.
7. Wei F-C, Mardini S. Flaps and reconstructive surgery. 2nd ed. Elsevier; 2017. p. 828.
8. Sieg P, Jacobsen HC, Hakim SG, Hermes D. Superficial ulnar artery: curse or blessing in harvesting fasciocutaneous forearm flaps. Head Neck. 2006;28(5):447–52. https://doi.org/10.1002/hed.20367.
9. Cavalheiro CS, Filho MR, Pedro G, Caetano MF, Vieira LA, Caetano EB. Clinical repercussions of Martin-Gruber anastomosis: anatomical study. Rev Bras Ortop. 2016;51(2):214–23. https://doi.org/10.1016/j.rboe.2016.02.003.
10. Li KK, Salibian AH, Allison GR, et al. Pharyngoesophageal reconstruction with the ulnar forearm flap. Arch Otolaryngol Head Neck Surg. 1998;124(10):1146–51. https://doi.org/10.1001/archotol.124.10.1146.
11. Huang AT, Day TA. Double paddle ulnar perforator free flap in reconstruction of through-and-through and fistulous defects of the head and neck. Laryngoscope. 2017;127(6):1302–5. https://doi.org/10.1002/lary.26440.
12. Thiem DGE, Siegberg F, Römer P, et al. Long-term donor site morbidity and flap perfusion following radial versus ulnar forearm free flap-a randomized controlled prospective clinical trial. J Clin Med. 2022;11(13) https://doi.org/10.3390/jcm11133601.

Vessel-Depleted Neck

36

Dustin A. Silverman and Chad A. Zender

History

- Patients who require microvascular free tissue reconstruction may present with some degree of a vessel-depleted neck (VND) in 7–52% of cases [1].
- No definitive algorithm for recipient vessel selection in the VDN currently exists; strategies are largely based on limited cohort studies and individual surgeon experience [2].
- Common arterial options: external carotid artery, internal mammary artery, transverse cervical artery, supraclavicular artery, thoracoacromial artery and branches, and superficial temporal artery.
- Common venous options: cephalic vein, internal mammary vein, vein grafts, and Corlett loops.
- Flap considerations are also critical. Donor sites with similar tissue components exist, each with varying pedicle lengths, which may influence flap selection for a particular defect with limited vascular options.

D. A. Silverman · C. A. Zender (✉)
Department of Otolaryngology- Head and Neck Surgery, University of Cincinnati Medical Center, Cincinnati, OH, USA
e-mail: zendercd@ucmail.uc.edu

Preoperative Care

- Detailed history and physical examination is critical to determine availability of reconstructive options.
- At both of the proposed donor and recipient sites, assess for the presence of scars or anatomic deformities from prior surgeries or injuries, postradiation changes to the neck or chest, external jugular vein patency, and presence of surgical devices that may preclude the use of arteriovenous options (e.g., implantable cardioverter–defibrillators, chemotherapy ports, central venous catheters).
- Modifiable risk factors such as tobacco and alcohol cessation, nutrition optimization, hyperglycemia, and hypothyroidism should ideally be addressed prior to intervention, particularly in non-oncologic cases (e.g., osteoradionecrosis) in order to maximize reconstructive success.
- Imaging.
  - Duplex ultrasonography (US) may be considered but provides less detail than contrast-enhanced axial or three-dimensional imaging techniques.
  - Single-phase computed tomography (CT) or magnetic resonance (MR) angiography may reveal the presence of arterial flow and tumor involvement of locoregional vessels.
  - Dual-phase CTA or multiphase MRA (similar to conventional angiography) captures

R. Rezaee, A. Tamaki (eds.), *Local, Regional, and Free Flaps for Head and Neck Reconstruction*,
https://doi.org/10.1007/978-3-032-03211-9_36

a delayed set of images to detail the patency of both arterial and venous structures [3].
- Prepare backup options and contingency plans in the highly challenging VDN scenario.

Flap and Vessel Selection

- Similar to microvascular reconstruction in the primary treatment setting, the ideal recipient vessel in the VDN should be accessible, anatomically predictable, and of adequate caliber with appropriate match to donor vasculature.
- "Out of field" vessels with minimal/no prior treatment are preferred, when applicable.
- Dissection should avoid sacrifice of additional reconstructive options.
- Contralateral neck.
  - When recipient vessels in the ipsilateral neck are not available or heavily treated, the use of vessels in the untreated contralateral neck should be strongly considered.
  - The contralateral facial and superior thyroid artery are most commonly utilized.
  - In some select patients, the contralateral transverse cervical vessels can be distally dissected to increase length and then reflected to or near midline for use.
  - The contralateral facial vein, internal jugular vein, and external jugular vein are accessible venous options.
  - Flap success rates that employ recipient vessels in the contralateral neck have been reported in excess of 95% [4].
- Use of a prior arterial anastomosis.
  - Flap anastomosis to a previously used recipient artery may be considered in select circumstances.
  - Studies demonstrate neovascularization develops within 7–10 days postoperatively, at which point division of a vascular pedicle may be feasible; however, flap survival is more probable when pedicle ligation occurs after postoperative day 12 [5, 6].
  - Caution should be maintained as total flap loss following division of a prior vascular pedicle as many as 3 years postoperatively has been reported [7]. This is particularly important when considering osseous flaps. These results suggest significant dominant blood supply via prior anastomotic vessels as many as 1–3 years after surgery.
- Free flap selection.
  - Selection of a fasciocutaneous or composite osteocutaneous flap with adequate pedicle length to reach recipient vessels is paramount. Pedicle geometry must also be considered in addition to vessel diameter.
    - Soft tissue flaps with longest pedicle lengths: radial forearm, anterolateral thigh, latissimus dorsi, rectus abdominus.
    - Osteocutaneous flaps with longest pedicle lengths: osteocutaneous radial forearm, fibula, scapular tip.
  - Reverse-flow scapula osteocutaneous flap [8].
    - Additional pedicle length may be achieved with the scapula free flap by harvesting the thoracodorsal artery.
    - Distal end of the thoracodorsal artery is anastomosed to recipient vessels. This allows reverse arterial flow into the flap via the circumflex scapular artery.
    - Notably, the presence of valves prevents reverse flow through accompanying venae. Vein grafts may be required to lengthen the venous pedicle. In many patients, the thoracodorsal vein is of suitable quality and caliber to be harvested, reversed and used as the donor vein.
- Surgical alternatives.
  - Utility of locoregional flaps should be considered prior to the use of a free flap in the setting of a VDN or necks described as being "toxic" due to anatomy and tissue quality from prior treatment.
  - Pectoralis major (PM), deltopectoral, trapezius, and latissimus dorsi flaps are traditional myo- and fasciocutaneous options and remain highly effective in the salvage setting [9].
  - Additional locoregional options such as the submental island, cervicofacial, supraclavicular, infraclavicular, deltopectoral, and temporalis flap are also commonly described.

Arterial Considerations

External Carotid Artery

Indications and Benefits

- External carotid artery (ECA) branches are most commonly utilized but may not be available in the VDN.
- In cases where the facial or superior thyroid arteries are not useable, the lingual artery and superficial temporal artery may be considered.
  - The lingual artery can also be suitable for use with retrograde flow from the tongue side if the ipsilateral external carotid is not suitable for dissection due to treatment and scarring effect. Dividing and testing the back flow can be considered.
  - An intact contralateral lingual artery must be present before using the lingual artery in the VDN.
- Though less commonly used, the occipital artery may be considered for radical parotidectomy and larger lateral cutaneous defects.
- The ECA itself is a larger caliber, high-pressure vessel with robust and reliable flow.
  - ECA may be harvested at its distal end with an end-to-end anastomosis to the flap pedicle.
  - The use of the ECA as a recipient artery may be safely used even when previous reconstructions are anastomosed to proximal ECA branches [10].
  - End-to-side anastomosis into the external carotid system can also be considered.

Anatomy

- Originates from the carotid bulb at the level of the superior border of the thyroid cartilage.
- Ascends deep to the posterior belly of the digastric muscle and posteromedial to the ramus of the mandible.
- Enters into the parotid gland parenchyma and bifurcates into its terminal branches (internal maxillary artery, superficial temporal artery).
- Proximal ECA internal vessel diameter reported to be 4.0 ± 0.6 mm and 2.85 ± 0.4 mm distally [11]. Thus, the distal (rather than proximal) ECA is typically selected given improved caliber match to flaps with smaller donor vessels (e.g., lateral arm free flap).

Pitfalls and Complications

- First-bite syndrome.
- Hypoglossal nerve injury.
- Facial nerve injury.
- Tongue ischemia with insufficient contralateral lingual artery flow.
- Atherosclerosis and luminal narrowing from prior radiation therapy.
- Unfavorable vessel caliber match to donor pedicle.

Operative Procedure

1. Utilize a preexisting transverse neck incision, when able.
2. Excise the submandibular gland.
3. Identify and protect the hypoglossal nerve as it courses over the ECA and deep to the internal jugular vein (IJV).
4. Divide the posterior belly of the digastric and stylohyoid muscles to identify the ECA deep to the digastric sling. Division of the digastric muscle may be avoided if additional artery length is not required, and potential vessel mismatch is not a factor.

   * In previously treated necks, it may be difficult to discern the hypoglossal nerve from the digastric tendon, so care and confirmation are critical.
5. Mobilize the ECA via dissection of the artery superiorly, deep, and posterior to the mandibular ramus. Ligate remaining ECA branches as required.
6. Additional ECA length is achieved by lifting the parotid tail off the sternocleidomastoid (SCM) muscle and dividing the ECA at its entry into the gland parenchyma.

   * Distal and superior ECA dissection is limited by the facial nerve.

   * Perform gentle, blunt dissection as needed along the superficial aspect of the ECA as it enters the parotid gland; this may prevent the need for meticulous facial nerve dissection and resultant injury.

Transverse Cervical Artery

Indications and Benefits

- Location in supraclavicular fossa at base of level IV renders the transverse cervical artery (TCA) less prone to injury from previous head and neck surgery and radiation effects.
- Useful in the primary and salvage laryngectomy setting with adequate distance from potential salivary fistula locations.
- Viable option in the event of carotid artery sacrifice (derived from thyrocervical trunk as it branches from the subclavian artery).

Anatomy

- Typically originates from the thyrocervical trunk 2.0 cm above the clavicle.
  - Variable origin from thyrocervical trunk, subclavian artery, and internal mammary artery (IMA) in 77%, 21%, and 2% of cases, respectively [12].
- Courses posterior and laterally over the scalene muscles toward the trapezius muscle.
- Mean internal vessel diameter of 2.6 mm with usable artery length of 2.0–4.0 cm [13].
- Accompanying transverse cervical vein may also have variable course either deep (75%) or superficial (25%) to the omohyoid muscle before draining into terminal portion of the external jugular vein or subclavian vein.

Pitfalls and Complications

- Previous injury or ligation from prior level IV neck dissection.
- May prevent the use of future ipsilateral supraclavicular artery island flap (nutrient supraclavicular artery typically arises from the TCA; however, may infrequently arise from the suprascapular artery).
- Phrenic nerve injury.
- Chyle leak.
- Pneumothorax.

Operative Procedure

1. Perform transverse neck incision or inferolateral incision extending over the SCM muscle to the clavicle.
2. Reflect SCM medially and trace posterior belly of the omohyoid muscle.
3. Identify TCA within the level IV adipofascial tissue deep and superior to the omohyoid. Avoid injury to the phrenic nerve inferior and deep to the plane of the TCA.
4. Dissect TCA proximally toward the thyrocervical trunk and distally/cephalad to increase length. If dissected distally and posteriorly under the trapezius for extra length through same or an extended incision, can reach the ipsilateral neck or past midline to reach the contralateral neck in some instances.

Internal Mammary Artery

Indications and Benefits

- One of the most commonly utilized arterial option in the VDN [2].
- Internal mammary artery (IMA) used extensively for coronary artery bypass grafting (CABG) given its resistance to atherosclerosis and large caliber with reliable flow.

Anatomy

- Originates from subclavian artery deep to clavicle.
- Descends from cephalad to caudad within anterior chest cavity.
- Courses inferiorly along the undersurface of the costal cartilages of the upper six ribs before bifurcating into terminal vessels (e.g., musculophrenic and superior epigastric arteries).
- Located approximately 1.5 cm lateral to the lateral border of the sternum.
- Traditionally harvested on *right* side as tends to be larger. Most ideal location within the third intercostal space where intraluminal caliber ranges from 1.9 to 2.6 mm [14].
- Reported to reach height of mandibular angle in 85% of cases [15].

Pitfalls and Complications

- Pneumothorax.
- Cosmetic chest wall deformity/depression.
- Prevents future CABG option.
- Reduced sternal blood supply.
- Intercostal nerve injury or neuralgia.

- A rib-sparing technique may also be used, but this decreases available length as the vessels are not fully released from their native location [16].

Operative Procedure

1. Perform vertical incision 1–2 cm lateral to the lateral sternal border from clavicle to third intercostal space.
2. Expose and divide medial aspect of the pectoralis major (PM) muscle to reveal the costal cartilages.
3. Exercise caution when dividing pectoralis muscle as perforating IMA branches will course through the muscle.
4. Trace IMA perforators to the anterior chest wall until the IMA is identified along the undersurface of the sternum.
5. Sharply incise and circumferentially free the perichondrium of the second and third costal cartilages.
6. Remove costal cartilage with blunt rongeur to reveal the deep perichondrium; incise deep perichondrium to expose the IMA and venae.

   * Usually unnecessary to remove more than 3–4 cm of a single rib to achieve adequate harvest.
7. Remove costal cartilages of ribs 4–6 to gain additional vessel length. If access will allow, distal ribs can be left in situ and vessels meticulously dissected distally and delivered underneath intact ribs to gain length and minimize flail component of chest. Care must be taken not to violate the pleura.

   * IMA caliber decreases as the vessel descends before branching into terminal vessels at fifth or sixth intercostal space.

   * Removal of rib cartilage above the second intercostal space will not yield increased length as IMA courses deep to join the subclavian artery.
8. Internal mammary vein (IMV) accompanies IMA and is located medial to the artery, approximately 1 cm lateral to the sternal border (Fig. 36.1).

   * Intraluminal caliber averages 3.0 mm and becomes smaller as it descends inferiorly.

   * IMV is thin-walled and prone to injury.
9. Following vessel harvest, fill wound with saline or sterile water to observe for air bubbles, which may indicate violation of the lung or pleura.

   * In event of pneumothorax, placement of suction drain and thoracic surgery consult is recommended.

Thoracoacromial Artery

Indications and Benefits

- Typically lies outside of prior surgical and radiation zones.
- Provides a large internal vessel diameter and is consistently present.
- Beneficial in reconstruction of tracheoesophageal and pharyngocutaneous fistulae given proximity to these defects.
- In the setting of prior PM flap harvest, the pectoral branch may remain viable if appropriate time for neovascularization has occurred.

Anatomy

- Thoracoacromial trunk originates from the second part of the axillary artery.
- Divides into four main arterial branches: deltoid, pectoral, acromial, clavicular (Fig. 36.2).
- Pectoral branch (which supplies the PM muscle) is familiar to head and neck surgeons and runs along the deep surface of the muscle within a protective layer of adipofascial tissue.
  - Pectoral branch penetrates the clavipectoral fascia 6–10 cm lateral to the sternoclavicular joint [17].

Pitfalls and Complications

- Elimination of pectoralis major flap as future reconstructive option (pectoral branch of thoracoacromial axis supplies the PM muscle).

Operative Procedure

1. Perform curvilinear incision over the deltopectoral groove and extend incision medially, approximately two fingerbreadths below the clavicle.

   * Use caution when designing incision in order to preserve the deltopectoral flap as reconstructive option.
2. Dissect through the fibrofatty tissue of the deltopectoral groove to identify the cephalic

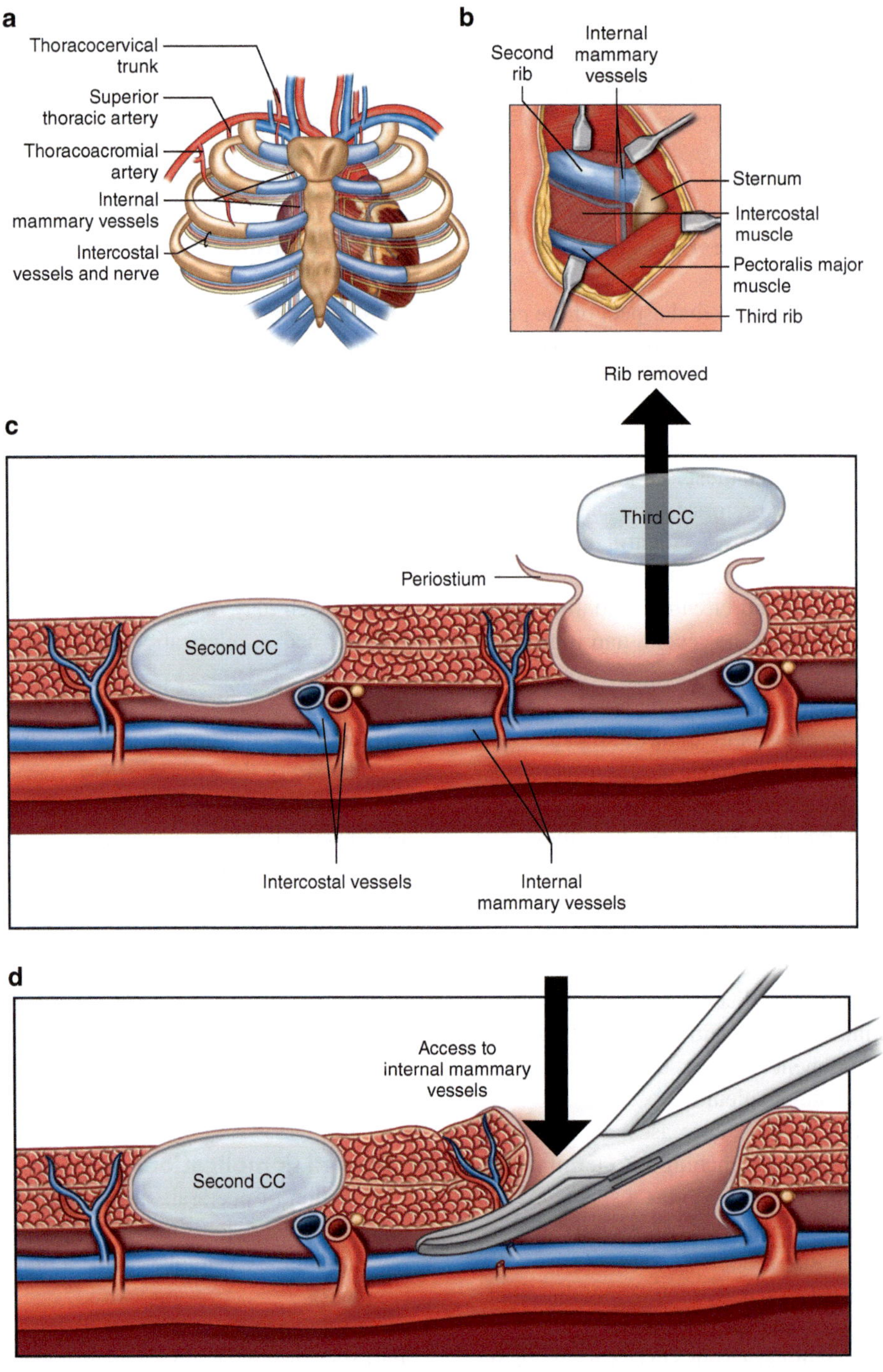

Fig. 36.1 Conventional technique for access to the internal mammary artery (IMA) and vein. (**a**) Normal neurovascular anatomy of the internal mammary artery and vein. (**b**) Schematic demonstrating the expected location of the IMA and vein following separation of the medial aspect of the pectoralis major muscle fibers; this allows access to the intercostal space between the second and third ribs. (**c**) Sagittal view of the internal mammary artery and vein. IMA perforators are traced to the anterior chest wall until the internal mammary artery is identified along the undersurface of the sternum. After sharply incising and circumferentially freeing the perichondrium of the third costal cartilage segment, the cartilage may be removed and allow access to the IMA. (d) Sagittal view of the internal mammary artery and vein. Further dissection of the intercostal muscles and perforators from the underlying internal mammary vessels

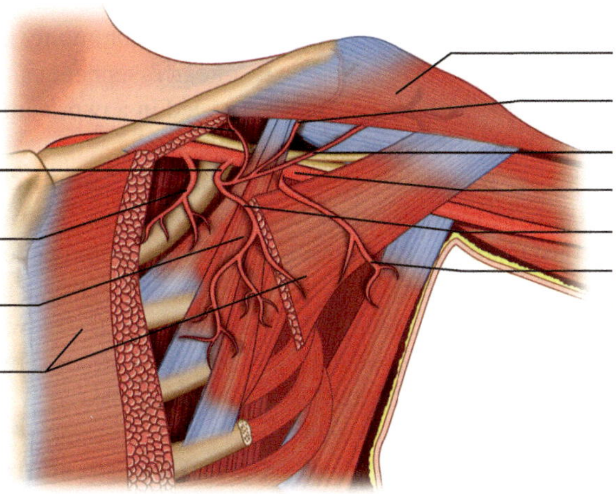

Fig. 36.2 Schematic of the thoracoacromial trunk arising from the second part of the axillary artery. Shown is the division of the thoracoacromial trunk and its division into the four main arterial branches: deltoid, pectoral, acromial, and clavicular

vein. The thoracoacromial axis may be identified parallel to the cephalic vein and slightly inferior within this tissue.

* If there is difficulty in identifying these vessels, consider division of the lateral attachments of PM muscle to the clavicle or split the muscle between its clavicular and sternal heads.

3. Identify deltoid artery as it courses between the PM and pectoralis minor muscles.
4. Continue dissection medially to identify the larger pectoral artery and thoracoacromial trunk.
5. Importantly, if the deltoid branch is of adequate size and length, the pectoral branch may be spared to preserve the PM flap. Otherwise, follow the pectoral branch inferiorly and dissect free from the PM until suitable caliber and length is achieved.
6. If the accompanying venae is not of sufficient quality, the cephalic vein may be easily accessed.

Venous Considerations

Cephalic Vein Transposition

Indications and Benefits

- Generally located outside of prior surgical and radiation zones.
- Reliable anatomy, superficial location, large caliber, and substantial available vessel length render this a highly useful option.
- Venous redundancy with the basilic and deep venous systems does not threaten upper extremity drainage.
- May be harvested proximally in combination with a thoracoacromial axis anastomosis or more distally into the forearm with transposition into the neck if additional length is required (especially useful with shorter flap pedicles).

Anatomy

- Long superficial vein that traverses the entire length of the upper extremity.
- Drains into the first part of the axillary vein.
- Courses between the brachioradialis and biceps brachii muscles of the forearm and then crosses superficial to the musculocutaneous nerve as it drains proximally in the groove of the lateral border of the biceps brachii.
- The vein continues to travel between the PM and deltoid muscles within the deltopectoral groove through the coracoclavicular (clavipectoral) fascia and into the axillary vein located deep to the junction of the middle and lateral thirds of the clavicle.

Pitfalls and Complications

- Inadvertent venous injury along its vessel length or proximally within the deltopectoral groove.
- Kinking of vein during transposition into the neck.

Operative Procedure

1. Perform incision just medial to the deltopectoral groove to avoid accidental venous injury.
2. Identify vein below subcutaneous fat as it courses along the deltopectoral groove.
3. Connect incision over the clavicle to the neck incision to enhance dissection and access.
4. Take care to avoid venous kinking during transposition into the neck.
5. Extent of distal dissection is dependent on length of vein required. Incision may be carried distally to the antecubital fossa.
6. Clip and divide branches along the length of the vein to increase mobilization.

Vein Graft

Indications and Benefits

- Used when additional vessel length is required.
- The external jugular vein or anterior jugular vein are easily accessible options.
- The cephalic vein and greater saphenous vein are also commonly harvested.
- Greater saphenous vein grafts may be harvested in a two-team fashion.

Pitfalls and Complications

- Thrombosis.
- Lower extremity edema.
- Ensure appropriate anterograde orientation of the vein graft. Flow in a retrograde direction may be obstructed by venous valves and result in thrombosis.

Operative Procedure

1. To harvest a greater saphenous vein graft, begin with an incision located proximal to the medial malleolus and 1–2 cm posterior to the edge of the tibia.
2. Incision may be lengthened to achieve appropriate length.
3. A stair-stepped incision approach may also be used.
4. Clip and divide small branches along the length of the vein to increase mobilization.
5. Single venous interposition graft may be anastomosed in an end-to-end fashion to either the artery or vein; however, longer grafts may be harvested to bridge gaps between both the arterial and venous vasculature.

Corlett Loop

Indications and Benefits

- Corlett loop, or arteriovenous fistula, is a variation of vein grafting (Fig. 36.3).
- May be considered when a useable locoregional artery and vein are not available.
- A long segment of the greater saphenous vein or cephalic vein is most commonly utilized in order to achieve both arterial and venous anastomoses.
- May be performed as a single-stage procedure in head and neck reconstruction [18].
- Usually considered a last-line procedure.

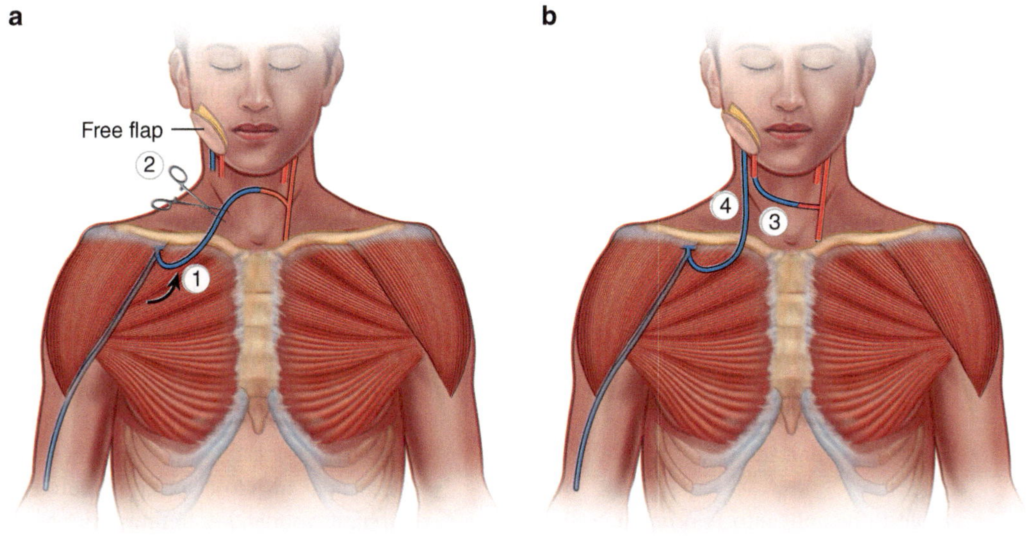

Fig. 36.3 Diagram of Corlett loop creation with free flap reconstruction. (**a**) (1) Cephalic vein of sufficient length is dissected and transposed to the contralateral external carotid artery or other external carotid artery branch to establish a temporary arteriovenous fistula (AVF). (2) Newly created arteriovenous loop fistula is divided at an appropriate length to allow for anastomosis to the flap artery and vein. (**b**) Final anastomotic pattern at the time of reconstruction. (3) The divided AVF is anastomosed to the free flap artery to achieve arterial flow. (4) Distal aspect of the previously transposed cephalic vein is anastomosed to the dominant free flap vena comitantes to achieve venous flow

Pitfalls and Complications

- Thrombosis.
- May require a two-stage procedure.
- Ensure appropriate anterograde orientation and flow of the graft.

Operative Procedure

1. Begin by harvesting a long segment of the greater saphenous vein or cephalic vein as described previously.
2. Anastomosis of the vein graft to an artery and vein in the base of the neck is then performed [19].
3. The newly created arteriovenous loop fistula may be utilized in a single stage and used immediately for anastomosis. Alternatively, the loop may be allowed to mature for 2 weeks prior to division.
4. Patient is placed on anticoagulation (typically protocols involving intravenous heparin and oral aspirin) during this period.
5. At the time of reconstruction, the arterial and venous limbs are then anastomosed to the flap artery and vein, respectively.

Neural Considerations

Indications and Benefits

- In the setting of a VDN, cranial nerves (commonly the trigeminal nerve and branches, facial, hypoglossal, and spinal accessory nerves) are often sacrificed to achieve complete oncologic resection [20].
- While primary nerve coaptation at the time of resection is not always performed, nerve defects may result in profound functional, sensory, and quality of life deficits.
  - If repair at the time of sacrifice is not possible, this should ideally be performed within 1 year prior to motor endplate degeneration (which completes near 2 years).
- When primary, tension-free neurorrhaphy is not possible, an interposition or “cable graft” should be used.
- Common donor nerves: Greater auricular, sural, nerve to vastus lateralis, medial or lateral antebrachial cutaneous.

- Greater auricular nerve.
  - Sensory nerve, routinely exposed during ablative cases.
  - Located parallel to and approximately 1.0 cm posterior to the external jugular vein.
  - Requires minimal additional dissection; commonly used interposition graft.
  - Should be avoided if oncologic concerns about involvement (e.g., parotid malignancies) are present.
- Sural nerve.
  - May be raised during fibula free flap harvest.
  - Serves as an additional cable graft option.
  - Able to be split into two or three divisions to accommodate multiple facial nerve branches [21].
  - Counsel patients regarding dorsal foot sensory deficits following harvest.
- Nerve to the vastus lateralis.
  - Motor nerve commonly used for facial nerve reconstruction during soft tissue and lateral skull base extirpation when facial nerve sacrifice is common.
  - Easily harvested as a vascularized nerve graft as this is exposed during dissection of the anterolateral thigh free flap pedicle.
  - Also accessible when harvested simultaneously with tensor fascia lata graft for static facial slings.
  - Up to 30 cm in length available with ideal caliber; arborizes into 3–6 nerve branches. Thus, workhorse for facial nerve reconstruction [22].
- Medial antebrachial cutaneous nerve.
  - Sensory nerve: provides sensory innervation to the medial, anteroulnar forearm, and skin overlying the olecranon.
  - Length in excess of 20 cm available with excellent donor match to facial nerve diameter and favorable branching pattern for multiple distal branches [23].
  - Most commonly arises from medial cord of the brachial plexus (80%), followed by the lower trunk of the brachial plexus (20%).
  - Originates in the axilla between the axillary artery and vein; travels distally within the arm along the basilic vein as it courses between the triceps brachii and brachialis muscles. Becomes superficial within the mid to distal arm where it then divides into an anterior and posterior branch at the level of the medial and lateral epicondyles [24].
- Lateral antebrachial cutaneous nerve.
  - Sensory nerve: provides sensory innervation to the lateral/radial half of the forearm.
  - Descends in close proximity to the cephalic vein and is commonly encountered central to slightly radial during radial forearm free flap harvest [25].
  - Located deep within the distal biceps muscle and tendon; pierces the deep fascia just proximal to the elbow joint where it then courses behind the cephalic vein before division into its anterior and posterior branches.

Pitfalls and Complications

- Synkinesis.
- Neuroma.
- Prolonged motor and sensory dysfunction at the recipient and donor sites.

Technical Considerations

- No current consensus regarding the use of motor versus sensory nerves for reconstruction.
- Polarity of nerve fibers during neurorrhaphy preparation should be considered.
  - Existing literature does not favor standard polarity over reversed polarity.
  - Animal models have demonstrated that reversed nerve grafts may reduce the risk of regenerating nerve fibers becoming "lost" at branch points [26].
  - Future studies are required to evaluate the impact of nerve polarity on regeneration, motor function, and sensation in head and neck reconstruction.

- Nerve conduits.
  - Construct used to span a gap between separate nerve endings to promote neuronal growth and regeneration.
  - Historically, autologous tissue including veins, arteries, and muscle have been employed.
  - Processed human acellular allogenic nerve grafts and xenografts are also available for bridging of larger gaps.
  - May obviate the need for additional donor site morbidity, decrease operating time, and lessen local tissue ingrowth.
  - Various synthetic nerve conduits are available.
    - *First generation*: polytetrafluoroethylene (ePTFE, Gore-Tex), non-resorbable silicone.
    - *Second generation*: polyglycolic acid (PGA), resorbable type I collagen, poly-DL-lactide-co-caprolactone, non-resorbable polyvinyl alcohol.
    - *Third generation*: experimental conduits designed to promote nerve regeneration through incorporation of neurotrophic factors, Schwann cells, and numerous other molecules [27].

Disclosure Statement No conflicts of interest to disclose.

References

1. Breik O, Praveen P, Parmar S. The vessel-depleted neck in head and neck microvascular reconstruction: extreme solutions for extreme situations. Curr Opin Otolaryngol Head Neck Surg. 2020;28(2):129–35. https://doi.org/10.1097/moo.0000000000000611.
2. Frohwitter G, Rau A, Kesting MR, Fichter A. Microvascular reconstruction in the vessel depleted neck – a systematic review. J Craniomaxillofac Surg. 2018;46(9):1652–8. https://doi.org/10.1016/j.jcms.2018.05.051.
3. Du E, Patel S, Huang B, Patel SN. Dual-phase CT angiography for presurgical planning in patients with vessel-depleted neck. Head Neck. 2019;41(9):2929–36. https://doi.org/10.1002/hed.25775.
4. Gschossmann JD, Balk M, Rupp R, et al. Results of contralateral anastomosis of microvascular free flaps in head and neck reconstruction. Ear Nose Throat J. 2022:1455613221112338. https://doi.org/10.1177/01455613221112338.
5. Kumar K, Jaffe W, London NJ, Varma SK. Free flap neovascularization: myth or reality? J Reconstr Microsurg. 2004;20(1):31–4. https://doi.org/10.1055/s-2004-818047.
6. Yoon AP, Jones NF. Critical time for neovascularization/angiogenesis to allow free flap survival after delayed postoperative anastomotic compromise without surgical intervention: a review of the literature. Microsurgery. 2016;36(7):604–12. https://doi.org/10.1002/micr.30082.
7. Moolenburgh SE, van Huizum MA, Hofer SO. DIEP-flap failure after pedicle division three years following transfer. Br J Plast Surg. 2005;58(7):1000–3. https://doi.org/10.1016/j.bjps.2005.04.040.
8. Zevallos JP, Urken ML. Reverse-flow scapular osteocutaneous flap for head and neck reconstruction. Head Neck. 2013;35(6):E171–4. https://doi.org/10.1002/hed.22914.
9. Chang BA, Asarkar AA, Horwich PM, Nathan CAO, Hayden RE. Regional pedicled flap salvage options for large head and neck defects: the old, the new, and the forgotten. Laryngoscope Investigat Otolaryngol. 2023;8(1):63–75. https://doi.org/10.1002/lio2.983.
10. Garg RK, Poore SO, Wieland AM, Sanchez R, Baskaya MK, Hartig GK. Recipient vessel selection in the difficult neck: outcomes of external carotid artery transposition and end-to-end microvascular anastomosis. Microsurgery. 2017;37(2):96–100. https://doi.org/10.1002/micr.22448.
11. Hiller A, Davis J, Schulz S, Henderson J, Wilhelmi BJ. Recipient vessel selection in head and neck reconstruction. Eplasty. 2017;17:e42.
12. Jacobson AS, Eloy JA, Park E, Roman B, Genden EM. Vessel-depleted neck: techniques for achieving microvascular reconstruction. Head Neck. 2008;30(2):201–7. https://doi.org/10.1002/hed.20676.
13. Tessler O, Gilardino MS, Bartow MJ, et al. Transverse cervical artery: consistent anatomical landmarks and clinical experience with its use as a recipient artery in complex head and neck reconstruction. Plast Reconstr Surg. 2017;139(3):745e–51e. https://doi.org/10.1097/prs.0000000000003085.
14. Canham PB, Finlay HM, Boughner DR. Contrasting structure of the saphenous vein and internal mammary artery used as coronary bypass vessels. Cardiovasc Res. 1997;34(3):557–67. https://doi.org/10.1016/s0008-6363(97)00056-4.
15. Morel F, Crampon F, Adnot J, Litzler PY, Duparc F, Trost O. Rerouting the internal thoracic pedicle: a novel solution for maxillofacial reconstruction in vessel-depleted situations? A preliminary anatomic study. Surg Radiol Anat. 2018;40(8):911–6. https://doi.org/10.1007/s00276-017-1965-1.
16. Jacobson AS, Smith M, Urken ML. Internal mammary artery and vein as recipient vessels in head and neck reconstruction. JAMA Otolaryngol Head Neck

Surg. 2013;139(6):623–8. https://doi.org/10.1001/jamaoto.2013.3062.
17. Davies MJ, van der Rijt R, Haddad R, Southwell-Keely J. The thoracoacromial axis in salvage head and neck reconstructive surgery, a case series. Case Reports Plast Surg Hand Surg. 2022;9(1):165–8. https://doi.org/10.1080/23320885.2022.2094270.
18. Ethunandan M, Cole R, Flood TR. Corlett loop for microvascular reconstruction in a neck depleted of vessels. Br J Oral Maxillofac Surg. 2007;45(6):493–5. https://doi.org/10.1016/j.bjoms.2006.08.014.
19. Moubayed SP, Giot JP, Odobescu A, Guertin L, Harris PG, Danino MA. Arteriovenous fistulas for microvascular head and neck reconstruction. Plast Surg (Oakv). 2015;23(3):167–70. https://doi.org/10.4172/plastic-surgery.1000925.
20. Hoshal SG, Solis RN, Bewley AF. Nerve grafts in head and neck reconstruction. Curr Opin Otolaryngol Head Neck Surg. 2020;28(5):346–51. https://doi.org/10.1097/moo.0000000000000649.
21. Lee MC, Kim DH, Jeon YR, et al. Functional outcomes of multiple sural nerve grafts for facial nerve defects after tumor-ablative surgery. Arch Plast Surg. 2015;42(4):461–8. https://doi.org/10.5999/aps.2015.42.4.461.
22. Revenaugh PC, Knott D, McBride JM, Fritz MA. Motor nerve to the vastus lateralis. Arch Facial Plast Surg. 2012;14(5):365–8. https://doi.org/10.1001/archfacial.2012.195.
23. Haller JR, Shelton C. Medial antebrachial cutaneous nerve: a new donor graft for repair of facial nerve defects at the skull base. Laryngoscope. 1997;107(8):1048–52. https://doi.org/10.1097/00005537-199708000-00008.
24. Ballard T, Smith T. Anatomy, medial antebrachial cutaneous nerve. *StatPearls*. StatPearls Publishing Copyright © 2023, StatPearls Publishing LLC.; 2023.
25. Boutros S, Yuksel E, Weinfeld AB, Alford EL, Netscher DT. Neural anatomy of the radial forearm flap. Ann Plast Surg. 2000;44(4):375–80. https://doi.org/10.1097/00000637-200044040-00004.
26. Roberts SE, Thibaudeau S, Burrell JC, Zager EL, Cullen DK, Levin LS. To reverse or not to reverse? A systematic review of autograft polarity on functional outcomes following peripheral nerve repair surgery. Microsurgery. 2017;37(2):169–74. https://doi.org/10.1002/micr.30133.
27. Gaudin R, Knipfer C, Henningsen A, Smeets R, Heiland M, Hadlock T. Approaches to peripheral nerve repair: generations of biomaterial conduits yielding to replacing autologous nerve grafts in Craniomaxillofacial surgery. Biomed Res Int. 2016;2016:3856262. https://doi.org/10.1155/2016/3856262.

Index

R. Rezaee, A. Tamaki (eds.), *Local, Regional, and Free Flaps for Head and Neck Reconstruction*,
https://doi.org/10.1007/978-3-032-03211-9

GPSR Compliance

The European Union's (EU) General Product Safety Regulation (GPSR) is a set of rules that requires consumer products to be safe and our obligations to ensure this.

If you have any concerns about our products, you can contact us on ProductSafety@springernature.com

In case Publisher is established outside the EU, the EU authorized representative is:

Springer Nature Customer Service Center GmbH
Europaplatz 3
69115 Heidelberg, Germany

Batch number: 10731395

Printed by Printforce, the Netherlands